STATISTICS *for*
EVIDENCE-BASED
PRACTICE
in NURSING

The Pedagogy

Statistics for Evidence-Based Practice in Nursing drives comprehension through various strategies that meet the learning needs of students, while also generating enthusiasm about the topic. This interactive approach addresses different learning styles, making this the ideal text to ensure mastery of key concepts. The pedagogical aids that appear in most chapters include the following:

Chapter Objectives

These objectives provide instructors and students with a snapshot of the key information they will encounter in each chapter. They serve as a checklist to help guide and focus study. Objectives can also be found within the book's online resources.

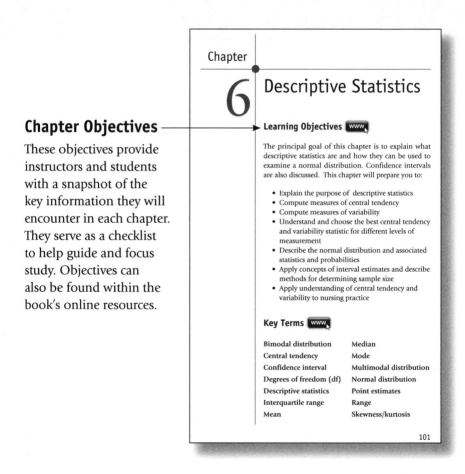

Chapter

6 Descriptive Statistics

Learning Objectives www

The principal goal of this chapter is to explain what descriptive statistics are and how they can be used to examine a normal distribution. Confidence intervals are also discussed. This chapter will prepare you to:

- Explain the purpose of descriptive statistics
- Compute measures of central tendency
- Compute measures of variability
- Understand and choose the best central tendency and variability statistic for different levels of measurement
- Describe the normal distribution and associated statistics and probabilities
- Apply concepts of interval estimates and describe methods for determining sample size
- Apply understanding of central tendency and variability to nursing practice

Key Terms www

Bimodal distribution	Median
Central tendency	Mode
Confidence interval	Multimodal distribution
Degrees of freedom (df)	Normal distribution
Descriptive statistics	Point estimates
Interquartile range	Range
Mean	Skewness/kurtosis

101

Key Terms `www`

Enter method	Percentage of variance
Goodness of fit	Predictor variable
Hierarchical method	R-square
Linearity	Regression model
Logistic regression	Residual
Method of least squares	Stepwise method
Multicollinearity	

INTRODUCTION

We have learned that correlations tell us whether variables of interest are related or associated with one another, and if so, how strong the relationship is. For example, a correlation coefficient of +.50 tells us that the variables are positively and moderately related to each other. Correlations and their strength provide important information about clinical phenomena that we are just beginning to explore. In correlation, we do not specify which are the independent and dependent variables, and all we are interested in is whether or not the variables are related. However, understanding how variables are related is usually a precursor to a more important level of understanding: prediction of the dependent variable by one or more independent variables.

Let us consider a study examining the relationship between fat and protein in the human body, and the correlation coefficient indicated that fat and protein are negatively related (i.e., protein level will increase as fat content decreases in the human body). Depending upon how strong the relationship is, we could then the value of one variable using the value of t case, does the level of protein predict the leve tion? Obviously, the estimation or predictio when the relationship is stronger. This is what

In clinical practice and research it is often n that a relationship exists between variables. how much influence is exerted by the indeper pendent variable—in other words, we want t

Key Terms

Found in a list at the beginning of each chapter, these terms will create an expanded vocabulary. Use the access code in the front of this book to access additional resources online.

Missing data occurs when a subject does not provide responses to a variable, data are skipped in data entry, or when a researcher found no way of measuring a variable. We need to pay careful attention to the pattern of missing data, as nonrandom missing data is a more serious problem than random missing data. In general, the problem gets worse as the amount of missing data increases. Missing data can be handled through either deletion or estimation. Deletion should be done only if the amount of missing data is small and it is missing in a random pattern. Otherwise, missing data should be estimated.

Outliers are another important source of errors in data and are defined as any unusual data value in the data set. Outliers can be spotted through visual displays like scatterplots or by transforming the raw data into z-scores. Outliers can be handled through deletion, transformation, or changing the score. Deletion should be done only if you have a sound reason to do so; otherwise transformation should be performed. If transformation does not solve the problem, you should consider changing the score.

All parametric tests require some assumptions to be met. Common assumptions include normality of the data, independence of the data, interval data, and the equality of variance. These assumptions should be checked before the data analysis is performed, as violations of the assumptions can distort the results.

Critical Thinking Questions

Review key concepts from each chapter with these questions at the end of each chapter. Complete these questions online and submit your answers directly to your instructor.

Critical Thinking Questions `www`

1. Why should the researcher examine the data before conducting data analysis? Explain.
2. Where would information about the treatment of missing data be found in a report of research?
3. Suppose that one of the collected variables was "Birth Year" and we found out that one of the respondents wrote down the current year instead of his actual year of birth. What seems to be an appropriate action for this data?
4. Use the data file called *satisfaction.sav* (found on the Student Companion Website using the access code card from the front of this text), and see which transformation method seems the most reasonable approach with an outlier(s).

Results: Unit response rates varied from 6% to 100%. Together, variability in understanding communication and capacity utilization were predictive of 27% of the variance in ventilator-associated pneumonia. Timeliness of communication was inversely related to pressure ulcers ($r = -0.38$; $P = .06$).

Conclusions: Not all elements of communication were related to the selected adverse outcomes. The connection between characteristics of the practice environment at the unit level and adverse outcomes remains elusive.

Self-Quiz

Test your knowledge of key concepts with these quick quizzes at the end of each chapter. Access these quizzes online using the code in the front of this book.

Self-Quiz www

1. Which of the following correlation coefficients represents the strongest relationship?
   a. $+.14$
   b. $+.82$
   c. $-.02$
   d. $-.34$
   e. $+.56$
2. True or false: If a correlation coefficient is -1.00, it means that the two variables will move in opposite directions with an equal unit change.
3. True or false: The correlation coefficient between age and depression is $+.85$. Since this coefficient is high enough, one can conclude that aging will cause increasing depression.

REFERENCES

Burtson, P. L., & Stichler, J. F. (2010). Nursing work environment and nurse caring: Relationship among motivational factors. *Journal of Advanced Nursing, 66*(8), 1819–1831. doi: 0.1111/j.1365-2648.2010.05336.x

Manojlovich, M., Antonakos, C. L., & Ronis, D. L. (2009). Intensive care units, communication between nurses and physicians, and patient's outcomes. *American Journal of Critical Care, 18*(1), 21–30.

Mor, V., Intrator, O., Feng, Z., & Grabowski, D. C. (2010). The revolving door of rehospitalization from skilled nursing facilities. *Health Affairs, 29*(1), 57–64.

STATISTICS *for* EVIDENCE-BASED PRACTICE *in* NURSING

MYOUNGJIN KIM, PHD
Assistant Professor
Mennonite College of Nursing
Illinois State University
Normal, Illinois

CAROLINE MALLORY, PHD, RN
Associate Dean of Research
Coordinator, Graduate Program
Professor
Mennonite College of Nursing
Illinois State University
Normal, Illinois

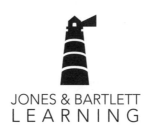

JONES & BARTLETT
LEARNING

World Headquarters
Jones & Bartlett Learning
5 Wall Street
Burlington, MA 01803
978-443-5000
info@jblearning.com
www.jblearning.com

Jones & Bartlett Learning books and products are available through most bookstores and online booksellers. To contact Jones & Bartlett Learning directly, call 800-832-0034, fax 978-443-8000, or visit our website, www.jblearning.com.

Substantial discounts on bulk quantities of Jones & Bartlett Learning publications are available to corporations, professional associations, and other qualified organizations. For details and specific discount information, contact the special sales department at Jones & Bartlett Learning via the above contact information or send an email to specialsales@jblearning.com.

Statistics for Evidence-Based Practice in Nursing is an independent publication and has not been authorized, sponsored, or otherwise approved by the owners of the trademarks or service marks referenced in this product.

Some images in this book feature models. These models do not necessarily endorse, represent, or participate in the activities represented in the images.

The screenshots in this product are for educational and instructive purposes only. All trademarks displayed are the trademarks of the parties noted therein. Such use of trademarks is not an endorsement by said parties of Jones & Bartlett Learning, its products, or its services, nor should such use be deemed an endorsement by Jones & Bartlett Learning of said third party's products or services.

The authors, editor, and publisher have made every effort to provide accurate information. However, they are not responsible for errors, omissions, or for any outcomes related to the use of the contents of this book and take no responsibility for the use of the products and procedures described. Treatments and side effects described in this book may not be applicable to all people; likewise, some people may require a dose or experience a side effect that is not described herein. Drugs and medical devices are discussed that may have limited availability controlled by the Food and Drug Administration (FDA) for use only in a research study or clinical trial. Research, clinical practice, and government regulations often change the accepted standard in this field. When consideration is being given to use of any drug in the clinical setting, the health care provider or reader is responsible for determining FDA status of the drug, reading the package insert, and reviewing prescribing information for the most up-to-date recommendations on dose, precautions, and contraindications, and determining the appropriate usage for the product. This is especially important in the case of drugs that are new or seldom used.

Production Credits

Executive Publisher: Kevin Sullivan
Acquisitions Editor: Amanda Harvey
Editorial Assistant: Sara Bempkins
Production Manager: Carolyn Rogers Pershouse
Marketing Communications Manager: Katie Hennessy
V.P., Manufacturing and Inventory Control: Therese Connell
Composition: Aptara®, Inc.

Cover Design: Scott Moden
Cover Images: clockwise from top left: © Digital Vision/Thinkstock; © Zen 2000/Dreamstime.com; © Wavebreak Media/Thinkstock; © Duncan Smith/Photodisc/Thinkstock; © Thinkstock Images/Comstock/Thinkstock
Printing and Binding: Edwards Brothers Malloy
Cover Printing: Edwards Brothers Malloy

To order this product, use ISBN: 978-1-4496-8669-7

Library of Congress Cataloging-in-Publication Data
Kim, MyoungJin.
  Statistics for evidence-based practice in nursing / MyoungJin Kim, Caroline Mallory.
      p. ; cm.
  Includes bibliographical references and index.
  ISBN 978-1-4496-4567-0 (pbk.) — ISBN 978-1-4496-8669-7
  I. Mallory, Caroline. II. Title.
  [DNLM: 1. Statistics as Topic–Nurses' Instruction. 2. Evidence-Based Nursing. 3. Nursing Research–methods. WA 950]
  610.73072—dc23
                                2012035550

6048
Printed in the United States of America
17 16 15 14 13   10 9 8 7 6 5 4 3 2

Dedication

• • •

To Darin, role model, best friend, and love of my life.

—Caroline Mallory

To Jiyoung, Kaleb, and Jacob, life-long partners and supporters of my life.

—MyoungJin Kim

• • •

Contents

Chapter

8 Getting Ready for the Analysis 157

Chapter

9 Examining Relationships Between and Among Variables 173

Chapter

10 Modeling Relationships 193

Preface

There is funny thing about email messages: sometimes they can surprise you. That was our sensation when we realized that Jones & Bartlett Learning had contacted us separately, but simultaneously, to determine our interest in writing a statistics textbook. Neither of us could have tackled this project alone, but together we were able to make some sense of nursing practice and statistics—at least that was our goal. You, the reader, will be the judge of our success.

As we discussed the possibility of writing a statistics book for nursing, we became more and more excited. We have found in our years of teaching research design, evidence-based practice (EBP), and statistics that many textbooks were available in each of the subjects, but none brought all of these perspectives together. We also found that students were often intimidated by the content and the technical language associated with the fields of research design, EBP, and statistics. It seemed important that any book we would write must be accessible and sensible, as well as integrate design, EBP, and statistics to create a truly useful resource.

This book may be useful for undergraduate students, but is really written for entry-level graduate students in Master of Science and Doctor of Nursing Practice programs. Many students entering these programs have not been working with research design, EBP, or statistics for quite some time, and these students may feel a sense of dread when told that such coursework is required in their program of study. We aim to put these students at ease with a reasoned explanation of the content in each chapter along with examples from nursing practice, research, and EBP, including step-by-step instructions on how to proceed with statistical analyses. We hope that this book will serve as a resource for nurses in advanced practice across a wide variety of settings and roles, from nurse executives to nurse practitioners. For more advanced students, this book will serve as a refresher on the basics of statistical analysis associated with research, evidence-based practice, and program evaluation.

Acknowledgments

We are deeply grateful to the editorial staff at Jones & Bartlett Learning for offering us this terrific opportunity. We also could not have accomplished this work without the sustained efforts of Dr. Susan Kossman and Dr. Robert Lynch, who dutifully pointed out all of our errors and confused writing, as well as making essential suggestions for improving the book. We are also in debt to the Master of Science students at Mennonite College of Nursing, Illinois State University, who reviewed the chapters and provided valuable feedback. Thanks also to our families for putting up with many late nights. Their love and support of us throughout this endeavor was great motivating force.

Reviewers

Karen Abate, PhD, RN, APRN
Assistant Professor
Notre Dame of Maryland University
Baltimore, MD

Kimberly Balko, MS, RN
Assistant Professor
Empire State College
Saratoga Springs, NY

Evelyn Brooks, RN, PhD
Professor
Missouri Western State University
St. Joseph, MO

Lynn B. Clutter, PhD, MSN, RN, BC, CNS, CNE
Assistant Professor, Langston
    University School of Nursing
Saint Francis Hospital,
    International Board Certified
    Lactation Consultant
Tulsa, OK

Rachel W. Cozort, PhD, MSN, RN
Assistant Professor of Nursing
Lenoir Rhyne University
Hickory, NC

Sherill Nones Cronin, PhD, RN-BC
Professor and Chair, Graduate
    Studies in Nursing
Bellarmine University
Louisville, KY

Rebecca J. Bartlett Ellis, PhD(c), MSN, RN
Clinical Assistant Professor
Indiana University School of
    Nursing at IUPUC
Indianapolis, IN

Mary Alice Hodge, PhD, RN
Director, BSN Programs
Gardner-Webb University
Boiling Springs, NC

Denise Hoisington, RN, MSN, PhD
Associate Professor
Ferris State University
Big Rapids, MI

Cheryl Kruschke, EdD, MS, RN
Assistant Professor
Regis University
Denver, CO

Janice L. O'Brien, PhD, RN,
  AHN-BC
Assistant Professor
Director, RN to BSN Program
Saint Peter's College
Jersey City, NJ

Catherine Pearsall, PhD, FNP, CNE
St. Joseph's College, Long Island
  Campus
Nursing Department
Patchogue, NY

Janet Philipp, EdD, RN
Professor and Chair, EdD Program
College of Saint Mary
Omaha, NE

Kathryn Reveles, DNP, RNC-NIC,
  CNS, CPNP-PC
Assistant Clinical Professor/Director
  PNP Concentrations
The University of Texas at El Paso
El Paso, TX

Beverly L. Roberts, PhD, FAAN
University of Florida
Gainesville, FL

Vicki M. Ross, RN, PhD
Adjunct Professor
University of Kansas School of
  Nursing
Kansas City, KS

Nancy A. Ryan-Wenger, PhD, RN,
  CPNP, FAAN
Director of Nursing Research
Nationwide Children's Hospital
Columbus, OH

Crystal C. Shannon, PhD, RN,
  MBA
Indiana University Northwest
Gary, IN

Ling Shi, PhD
Department of Nursing
University of Massachusetts, Boston
Boston, MA

Charlotte Ward, PhD, RN, CNE
Professor, Armstrong McDonald
  School of Nursing
College of the Ozarks
Point Lookout, MO

Priscilla Sandford Worral, PhD,
  RN
Upstate Medical University Health
  System
Syracuse, NY

Chapter

1

Evidence-Based Practice in Nursing, or Why Do I Need to Take Statistics?

Learning Objectives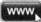

This chapter will introduce you to the rationale for advanced statistical preparation in nursing. Upon completing this chapter, you should be able to:

- Understand trends in health care and what these mean for evidence-based practice
- Define evidence-based practice as a foundation for nursing practice
- Describe different levels of evidence and how these are connected to statistics
- Understand the relevance of statistics for evidence-based practice in nursing

Key Terms

Efficacy

Evidence-based practice

Levels of evidence

Statistics

INTRODUCTION

As a nurse, you are accountable every day to your patients, your employer, and your profession to ensure that the quality of care you deliver is the best available. How will you be certain that your clients receive the best quality nursing care? Your professional experience and previous training, while important, are not sufficient to ensure confidence in the quality of nursing care. Over time, new knowledge and information become available, and your ability to engage in **evidence-based practice**, in which the selection of the most appropriate treatment, assessment approach, or evaluation technique are based on scientific review and hold the keys to providing high-quality nursing care.

We understand that **statistics** is an important tool of evidence-based practice, and if you are reading this book, we suspect that you are enrolled in a course or program of study that will help you to understand the application of statistics for evidence-based practice in nursing. We commend you for taking this important step to improve your competence and promote excellence in nursing care. As a nurse with advanced education in statistics and evidence-based practice, you will be well qualified to make important contributions to health care, nursing practice, and the well-being of patients across a variety of settings.

TRENDS SHAPING HEALTH CARE AND NURSING

We are entering a period of substantial change in health care. The passage and the initial implementation of federal healthcare reform in 2009–2010 through the Patient Protection and Affordable Care Act marked a shift toward more comprehensive insurance coverage for Americans. The profession of nursing has long supported movement toward universal health insurance coverage, as it is an important step in ensuring that patients are not overly burdened by out-of-pocket healthcare costs and are entitled to receive high-quality health care (American Nurses Association, 2008).

Particularly important to nurses in, or considering enrolling in, graduate programs is that healthcare reform is expanding insurance coverage for illness prevention and health promotion. One immediate consequence of this reform is the increased demand for primary care clinicians, such as nurse practitioners and midwives. Already, colleges and universities are seeing an increase in the number of applications to graduate programs in nursing to meet the needs in primary care. New graduates of these programs will be entering practice in a highly complex and dynamic healthcare system that is facing serious challenges.

Contributing to the complexity and challenges in health care is the increasing attention to quality and safety across settings. In 1999, the Institute of Medicine (IOM) released its landmark report *To Err Is Human* on the safety and quality of health care in the United States. The findings called attention to considerable problems within healthcare systems that lead to unacceptable levels of death and disability. In addition to the loss of life and reduced quality of life experienced by patients and their families, errors in diagnosis and treatment of patients result in cost overruns that contribute to the escalating cost of health care and insurance. The IOM report and subsequent work have resulted in very close scrutiny of safety and quality at all levels of the healthcare system, including nursing. For example, attention is turning to nursing-sensitive indicators of quality (Dunton & Montalvo, 2009). These include fall-related injuries, pressure ulcers, hospital-acquired infections, and others. Organizations such as The Joint Commission that inspect and accredit healthcare institutions are particularly interested in the quality of nursing care as measured by nursing-sensitive indicators. Thus, many hospitals and other institutions are updating and evaluating their protocols related to these indicators, which requires the skills of advanced practice nurses with training in the use of statistics and evidence-based practice.

What is the profession of nursing doing to address the concerns identified by the IOM and other bodies? There is strong evidence to suggest that patient outcomes in a variety of settings are related, in part, to the educational preparation of the nursing staff. Nurse researchers have found that educational preparation is a factor in morbidity and mortality rates. For example, Linda Aiken and colleagues (2003) found that as the ratio of baccalaureate nurses to patients rose, patient outcomes improved. There has long been strong evidence that advanced practice nurses, such as nurse practitioners, nurse midwives, and nurse anesthetists, provide care that leads to equivalent or better patient outcomes than physicians (Laurant et al., 2005). In 2010, the IOM released another report, *The Future of Nursing,* noting that the quality of health care in the United States is dependent upon the quality of nursing care.

The Future of Nursing outlines expectations for increasing the number of advanced practice nurses who provide primary care and facilitating nurses to practice to the full extent of their education. Inherent in these recommendations is the recognition of nurses' role in promoting safety and quality of patient care through evidence-based practice.

Recognizing the important role that advanced practice nurses have in the healthcare system, the American Association of Colleges of Nursing (AACN) has recommended that the Doctor of Nursing Practice (DNP) degree be the educational entry level for advanced practice nurses (2006). AACN understands that advanced practice nurses are expected to deliver a variety of skills that are not currently included in most master's degree curricula, including leadership and management, advanced evidence-based practice, and application of healthcare policy. The transition to the DNP as the entry level of training for advanced practice is controversial but is expected to take effect in 2015. At that time, the accrediting body for advanced practice programs, the Commission on Collegiate Nursing Education, will no longer review or accredit master's programs for advanced nursing practice, but will only consider for review DNP programs. Toward this expectation, we contend that nurses pursuing graduate education need a strong understanding of statistics to implement evidence-based practice. This book is designed to help nurses develop the skills necessary to carry out evidence-based practice.

Case Study

In 2008, Marian Racco, the ICU Clinical Coordinator, and Beverly Phillips, the Clinical Coordinator for Wound and Ostomy Care at Hunterdon Medical Center in New Jersey, were alarmed when an obese patient in the intensive care unit developed a stage III pressure ulcer. They determined that a better protocol for preventing pressure ulcers in that setting was required. They undertook an evidence-based practice project consisting of a thorough review of the evidence; this was used to design an improved protocol, which they then tested to determine if patients would have better skin outcomes. Using a descriptive study design, they collected data on 50 patients undergoing the protocol, with statistical analysis demonstrating positive outcomes for the majority of patients. The work of Racco and Phillips is a good example of how evidence-based practice can improve patient care.

EVIDENCE-BASED PRACTICE

Have you been a patient lately? What did you expect of the nurses who were providing your care? It is reasonable to expect that, for whatever intervention the nurse is carrying out, there should be some evidence to support the use of that intervention. Yet, it is only recently that we have begun to amass the volume of evidence needed to support particular nursing interventions. Dr. Mallory tells the following story.

> When I began my nursing career in 1985, it was common practice to treat pressure ulcers with all sorts of strange remedies. While working in nursing homes, I saw nurses apply heat lamps, antacids, and sugar to superficial and deep pressure ulcers. At that time, there was no research to investigate the efficacy of prevention or treatment interventions for pressure ulcers, and nurses were forced to rely on trial and error. Pressure ulcers are just the sort of problem that nurses care about, and through the accumulation of evidence we learned how pressure ulcers are formed, leading to prevention efforts and what treatments worked best to preserve and grow healthy tissue after an ulcer has formed. Now when we prescribe a prevention regimen to improve mobility, hydration, and nutrition, we know that evidence is backing up our efforts. Furthermore, we can educate our patients with the evidence, so they can be confident in the approach we have recommended. Our ability to combine evidence to meet a patient's individual needs and apply this information with a good dose of clinical judgment is what evidence-based practice is all about.

Evidence-based practice is clinical decision making using the best evidence available in the context of individual patient preferences by well-informed expert clinicians (Melnyk & Fineout-Overholt, 2005). There are many kinds of evidence that nurses can integrate into their practice (see **Figure 1-1**). We strive to use the best quality evidence available. Types of evidence range from our professional experience and expert opinion to proven theoretical propositions and findings from research. The volume and quality of evidence available depends on the nature of the clinical problem. From the earlier example, we know quite a bit about preventing pressure ulcers, but much less about the best way to encourage adherence to complex treatments of chronic illness. **Levels of evidence** are a useful way to think about what kinds of evidence are available, how these are connected to statistical tests, and what kinds of clinical questions each type of evidence can answer.

Let's examine the levels of evidence table (see **Table 1-1**). Keep in mind that the evidence table is similar to a healthy diet—that is, you need a bit of everything to have a good understanding of any given clinical situation or problem. Using our pressure ulcer example, we could ask a question like, "What is the patient experience of pain associated with a pressure ulcer?" Such a question would be best answered with evidence from descriptive studies in which researchers asked patients with a pressure ulcer about associated pain. On the other hand, if we wanted to know

Figure 1-1

Elements of evidence-based practice. *Source:* Adapted from Melnyk, B. M., & Fineout-Overholt, E. (2005). *Evidence-based practice in nursing and healthcare.* Philadelphia, PA: Lippincott Williams & Wilkins.

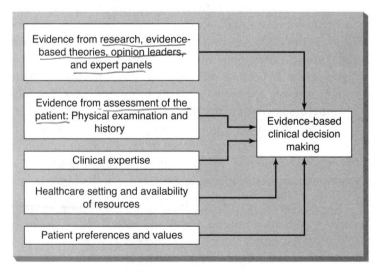

Table	
1-1	Levels of Evidence

Type of Research Evidence	Uses	Strength of the Evidence
Descriptive or exploratory research (single studies that report frequencies, averages, and variation)	Helps to answer questions about the nature of a problem (population or phenomenon being studied), such as "How many people are affected?" or "What is the subjective patient experience?"	Best evidence for describing problems or concerns in health care
Correlational research (single studies that report correlation coefficients such as Pearson's r)	Provides information about the relationship between factors, such as, "Is body weight related to the formation of pressure ulcers?"	Useful evidence for beginning to understand complex health problems
Comparative research (single studies that report on differences between groups using t-tests or ANOVA)	Helps to answer questions about how two or more groups are different on some factor, for example, "Does blood pressure vary between men and women?"	Evidence from these studies may be combined with correlational research to better describe the factors influencing health
Case controlled and cohort studies (single "natural experiments" that help us predict outcomes)	Provides information on what factors might influence or predict health outcomes, such as "Does smoking predict lung cancer?"	Strong preliminary evidence for examining cause and effect
Experimental or randomized controlled trials (single studies that test cause and effect)	Studies examine the effect of an intervention on patient outcomes. For example, "Does turning a patient every 2 hours prevent pressure ulcers?"	Very good evidence for examining cause and effect, especially the effect of interventions on patient outcomes

(continues)

Table	
1-1	Continued

Type of Research Evidence	Uses	Strength of the Evidence
Meta-analyses (analyses of existing randomized controlled trials to determine the effectiveness of interventions)	These studies combine many previous experiments on one or more interventions and their effects on a patient outcome to answer a question such as, "What do all of the studies on patient turning tell us about the effect on pressure ulcers?"	Strongest evidence for cause and effect and the effectiveness of an intervention

whether a wet-to-dry dressing or a hydrophilic dressing was the best for healing a pressure ulcer, evidence from randomized clinical trials comparing these two approaches would be the most useful. The nurse needs to skillfully interpret reports of research, including the statistical results, in order to determine the quality of the evidence and the applicability to any given clinical situation. Each type of research approach, exploratory to experimental, has its own statistical analyses that correspond to the kind of research question that is being asked and the type of data that has been collected. In this text we will restrict our discussion to quantitative research evidence. There are other valid forms of evidence such as expert opinion and findings from qualitative studies; however, since this text is focused on statistics and evidence-based practice, we will limit our discussion to approaches that use statistical methods for analyzing data.

STATISTICS AND EVIDENCE-BASED PRACTICE

Statistics are a useful tool for expressing data or characteristics in a scientific way. Going back to the earlier case study, let us assume that both wet-to-dry dressing and hydrophilic dressings were effective for healing a pressure ulcer with only a subtle difference in the healing rate. Such small differences may be difficult to observe in a single patient. We need to use the power of statistical analysis in combination with the right kind of study to determine if this subtle difference is an actual difference and not just luck or chance. The power of statistics to help us decide the effectiveness of a treatment is one aspect of how statistics are important in implementing evidence-based practice.

A statistician is a person who specializes in the application and/or development of statistical approaches for understanding data. While there are nurse statisticians, most nurses in advanced practice or leadership roles are not statisticians but are experts in their chosen field. However, nurses in advanced practice are still expected to be competent in the use of statistics for conducting evidence-based practice projects. The American Association of Colleges of Nursing (AACN, 2006) has specified that nurses at the DNP level should be able to do the following:

- Use analytic methods to critically appraise existing literature and other evidence to determine and implement the best evidence for practice.
- Design and implement processes to evaluate outcomes of practice, practice patterns, and systems of care within a practice setting, healthcare organization, or community against national benchmarks to determine variances in practice outcomes and population trends.
- Design, direct, and evaluate quality improvement methodologies to promote safe, timely, effective, efficient, equitable, and patient-centered care.
- Use research methods appropriately to:
  - collect relevant and accurate data to generate evidence for nursing practice
  - inform and guide the design of databases that generate meaningful evidence for nursing practice
  - analyze data from practice
  - design evidence-based interventions
  - predict and analyze outcomes
  - examine patterns of behavior and outcomes
  - identify gaps in evidence for practice

Each of the criteria listed above require quantitative and statistical reasoning skills. The AACN expectations for the DNP are well aligned with the rising expectations for graduate nurses in all settings as set forward by the *Future of Nursing* report from the IOM (2010).

CAROLINE'S STORY

I remember my first statistics course. I was so worried about my ability to learn the material that I set my goal at earning a "C" in the course. I kept telling myself "If I can just pass this class, then I won't have to worry about statistics again." Much to my surprise, I earned an "A" and found out that I was not stupid when it came to math or logical thinking—I just had not practiced enough. Most of us can remember a time when we were just learning a new skill, perhaps physical assessment or aseptic technique. Initially, we might have been quite clumsy or not understood completely the nuances of the skill. Statistics is just like that; a new skill that with practice becomes familiar and promotes in-depth understanding.

In our experience, nurses entering graduate programs are often unsure of their quantitative reasoning skills and have not practiced using statistics since their undergraduate or basic nursing program. As a nurse embarking on a more in-depth study of statistics and evidence-based practice, you may feel anxious about the current state of your skills. You may even question whether you *really* need additional training in statistics. Our objective in this book is to make statistics accessible and help you understand the importance of statistics to your practice. We hope that you are motivated to persevere in statistics to promote the quality and safety of patient care.

MYOUNGJIN'S STORY

I began my journey in statistics with a master's program. Being a business major previously, switching to statistics was not an easy transition. Over the years of statistical consulting, I have seen students who did not know where to go for help with statistical analysis for their data, and some who tried to be a self-learner but struggled with where to begin. They need a better and new way to resolve their problems. Through the use of evidence and my personal experience helping others, I hope that everyone will see the role of statistics in evidence-based nursing practice, understand statistics better, and become a competent clinician delivering the best quality of care.

SUMMARY

In this chapter, we have discussed some of the reasons that nurses need to develop skills for evidence-based practice, especially a strong understanding and use of statistics. Trends in healthcare policy and greater emphasis on quality and safety of patient care are resulting in a re-visioning of graduate nursing education to include an improved skill set in evidence-based practice. We learned that there are levels of research evidence that correspond to different types of research questions and that the strength of the evidence also varies accordingly. Nurses must be able to judge the quality of research evidence for use in practice, and understanding statistics helps us to do that. We also learned that the advanced practice nurse is more than just a consumer of research and statistics, but must also be competent in the use of statistics for evidence-based practice projects.

Critical Thinking Questions

1. Read the summary of the Institute of Medicine's report *To Err Is Human: Building a Safer Health System* (1999). What is the nurse's role in ensuring quality and safety?
2. Go to the American Association of Colleges of Nursing website and read the essentials for the Doctor of Nursing Practice (http://www.aacn.nche.edu/DNP/pdf/Essentials.pdf). What are your thoughts on the expectations for evidence-based practice for advanced practice nurses?
3. What do you think the role of statistics is in making evidence-based decisions?
4. On a scale of 0–10, with 10 being the most anxious, how would you rate your anxiety about statistics? What measures are you prepared to take to reduce your anxiety?

Self-Quiz

1. True or false: The Affordable Care Act provides for the expansion of insurance to cover more Americans.
2. True or false: The Institute of Medicine's report *To Err is Human* makes recommendations for nursing education and practice.

3. True or false: Evidence-based practice is best described as the use of only research for making clinical decisions.

4. True or false: Evidence from experimental research is best for describing the number of people affected by chronic disease.

5. True or false: Statistics is a scientific approach to express data or characteristics being studied.

6. True or false: Evidence-based practice is always founded on research evidence.

7. True or false: Nurses with master's and doctor of nursing practice degrees are expected to carry out original research.

REFERENCES

Aiken, L. H., Clarke, S. P., Cheung, R. B., Sloane, D. M., & Silber, J. H. (2003). Educational levels of hospital nurses and surgical patient mortality. *Journal of the American Medical Association, 290,* 1617–1623.

American Association of Colleges of Nursing (AACN). (2006). *The essentials of doctoral education for advanced nursing practice.* Retrieved from http://www.aacn.nche.edu/publications/position/DNPEssentials.pdf

American Nurses Association (ANA). (2008). *Health system reform agenda.* Retrieved from http://www.nursingworld.org/Content/HealthcareandPolicyIssues/Agenda/ANAsHealthSystemReformAgenda.pdf

Dunton, N., & Montalvo, I. (2009). *Sustained improvement in nursing quality: Hospital performance on NDNQI indicators, 2007–2008.* Silver Spring, MD: American Nurses Association.

Institute of Medicine (IOM). (1999). *To err is human: Building a safer health system.* Retrieved from http://www.iom.edu/~/media/Files/Report%20Files/1999/To-Err-is-Human/To%20Err%20is%20Human%201999%20%20report%20brief.pdf

Institute of Medicine (IOM). (2010). *The future of nursing: Leading change, advancing health.* Retrieved from http://www.iom.edu/Reports/2010/The-Future-of-Nursing-Leading-Change-Advancing-Health.aspx

Laurant, M., Reeves, D., Hermens, R., Braspenning, J., Grol, R. & Sibbald, B. (2005). Substitution of doctors by nurses in primary care [Review]. *The Cochrane Database of Systematic Reviews, 2.*

Melnyk, B. M., & Fineout-Overholt, E. (2005). *Evidence-based practice in nursing and healthcare.* Philadelphia, PA: Lippincott Williams & Wilkins.

2

Statistical Essentials I

Learning Objectives

The principal goal of this chapter is to provide you with an understanding of the basic statistical concepts essential for interpreting and performing statistical analyses. This chapter will prepare you to:

- Explain the general concepts of statistics and understand related terminology
- Distinguish sample from population
- Distinguish descriptive from inferential statistics
- Discuss random and nonrandom sampling procedures and explain the strengths and limitations of each procedure
- Discuss the application of sampling to inferential statistics and how this relates to evidence-based practice

Key Terms

Central tendency

Confidence level

Descriptive statistics

Hypothesis testing

Inferential statistics

Nonrandom sampling

Parameter

Population

Power analysis

Random sampling

Sample

Sampling

Sampling distribution

Sampling error

Variability

STATISTICS

What is statistics? Statistics is an empirical method for collecting, organizing, summarizing, and presenting data, and to make inferences about the population from which the data are drawn. Statistics is used extensively in many fields of study and it is important to ensure that statistics are appropriately applied to research and other quantitative forms of inquiry. One of the first steps in understanding and applying research to practice is learning the basic premises of statistics.

Most of us do not understand why we need to study statistics. In fact, you may dislike statistics or think that you will never use statistics. You may not know it, but you are living in a world full of statistics:

- Despite the current easing of the nursing shortage due to the recession, the U.S. nursing shortage is projected to grow to 260,000 registered nurses by 2025 (Buerhaus, Auerbach, & Staiger, 2009).
- Around 30% of people aged 65 years or older living in the community and more than 50% of those living in residential care facilities or nursing homes fall every year, and about 50% of those fall repeatedly (Baranzini et al., 2009).

These example statistics are not a matter of opinion or conjecture. Unlike everyday observation, researchers use the power of statistics to ensure that a study was designed carefully, and statistical findings are trustworthy.

Let us look at another example. Suppose you are shopping at a local grocery store and are used to paying $3.27 for a gallon of milk. One day, you find that a gallon of milk is priced at $20.00. You would be shocked and very likely would put the milk back on the shelf. You may not know it, but you just made a rational decision. A rational decision is based on the probability of whether an event is likely to occur; we do not take an action if the probability of an event is not likely. This differs from making an irrational decision, which may occur when we do not pay adequate attention or base our decision on incomplete information. The probability of an event occurring is a statistical concept.

There are many important essential concepts in statistics. In this text, you will learn how to comfortably understand and use statistical findings. In this chapter, we discuss some of the most important statistical essentials so that you can smoothly progress towards more complex topics and eventually use these tools as advanced practice nurses.

Population Versus Sample

A **population** is an entire group of individuals that a researcher wants to study. A **sample** is a subset of a population from which a researcher draws conclusions that are used to understand the population. For example, we are very interested in the prevention and treatment of diabetes, but it would be impossible to study every single diabetic person. Instead, we study a small group, perhaps 100 children aged 10–16 in order to speculate in a scientific way about all children aged 10–16 living with diabetes in the United States.

Occasionally, research is conducted on a population. One example of population-based research is the U.S. Census. In the census, all people residing in the United States are asked to complete the survey. However, in most health-related studies, researchers collect data from a sample that represents the population.

Numerical measurements taken from a population are **parameters**, and they are usually unknown. For instance, average job satisfaction of all nurses in the United States is a parameter when all nurses in the United States are defined as the population. On the other hand, those taken from a sample are statistics. For instance, job satisfaction of a selected group, or sample, of nurses in the United States is a statistic.

Descriptive and Inferential Statistics

Descriptive Statistics

Descriptive statistics are used to describe or convey an understanding of data. Consider a nursing college that wants to know more about the admission records of incoming nursing students. The college typically collects data on average age, entering grade point average, standardized test scores, and family income. The college will have to organize and summarize the data in order to understand the essential nature of the data, which would allow the college to know what characterizes the average student profile, especially when the number of data units is large. Descriptive statistics allow data to be organized, summarized, and described in a format that is more easily understood. Through descriptive statistics, administrators at the college will better understand the characteristics of students admitted to the college in a given year. For instance, the average student admitted to the college this year is 19 years old with a GPA of 3.89, a score of 24 on the ACT, and from families making $65,000 per year. Summarizing the data with descriptive statistics is a more efficient way to understand the student characteristics than having to examine every individual student record. With descriptive statistics, we can present the data with the use of graphs, charts, tables, and/or numerical measures such as **central tendency** and **variability**. We discuss descriptive statistics in more detail in Chapters 5 and 6.

Inferential Statistics

An inference is a conclusion based on logical reasoning in the absence of evidence or when only incomplete evidence is available. **Inferential statistics** allows a researcher to generalize the results from a sample to a population through **hypothesis testing**. Suppose you are hired by United States Department of Health and Human Services to examine how Americans feel about healthcare reform. You could survey every American on their opinion about the reform; however, this would be a costly and lengthy study with a likelihood that someone would be left out. Therefore, you take a sample of Americans, following a strategy to ensure that this sample accurately represents all Americans, ask their opinion about healthcare reform, draw conclusions from those data, and then infer those findings to the population. If you have been careful about sampling, we will have a good idea of what all Americans think about healthcare reform. We should note here that this inference process often relies on the representativeness of the sample for a given population. We discuss different sampling procedures in more detail in a later section of this text.

Inferential statistics help the practicing nurse make clinical treatment decisions or recommendations. What nurses often need to know is the strength or quality of the research evidence in support of a particular treatment or how various treatments compare with regard to effectiveness. Inferential statistics are tools to determine the strength of research evidence. For example, Seidel and colleagues (2008) conducted a meta-analysis (reviewing all randomized controlled trials and reanalyzing the combined data) on the effectiveness of antipsychotics for pain management. Across 770 participants in 11 studies, Seidel et al. found that antipsychotics were effective for pain management, but that extrapyramidal and sedation effects are a major consideration in prescribing. The advanced practice nurse may find this information important for treatment decisions but must be able to weigh the strengths and limitations of such work, including the applicability or generalizability of the study.

It may seem that descriptive statistics and inferential statistics are two separate functions. However, descriptive statistics allows you to examine the collected data and to explain it better. Therefore, researchers use descriptive statistics as a prerequisite step to the use of inferential statistics.

Sampling

So, why do we select a sample from a population? The answer is simple. In many cases, a population is too large and too costly to access as a whole. Therefore, we take a sample out of the population and try to infer what we find from sample to population.

The researcher must take care in his or her approach to sampling. Because inferences are made from sample to population, it is important that the sample is the best representation of the population, in that it resembles the population as much as possible. Without careful sampling, inferences may be flawed (see **Figure 2-1**). In the world of evidence-based practice, it is important that the nurse evaluates how representative the sample is and, equally important, if the sample reflects the target population. For example, if the nurse is treating a child, it will be important to examine evidence from studies with children with similar characteristics. Clinically and statistically, it is problematic to apply evidence from studies of adults to children.

Random Sampling

There are two types of **sampling** procedures: random sampling and nonrandom sampling. **Random sampling** is a method of selecting subjects based on chance alone and is the strongest approach to sampling. All random sampling procedures select subjects for a sample based on an equal chance of selection for each person. If a researcher wishes to draw a random sample of 10 from a population of 100, we would say that each person in the population has 10 chances in 100 of selection; each person has an equal chance of selection. Random sampling does require that the entire population is known and can be accessed for sampling, such as all patients over the age of 65 with suspected myocardial infarction admitted through the emergency room

Figure 2-1

Taking a sample from a population.

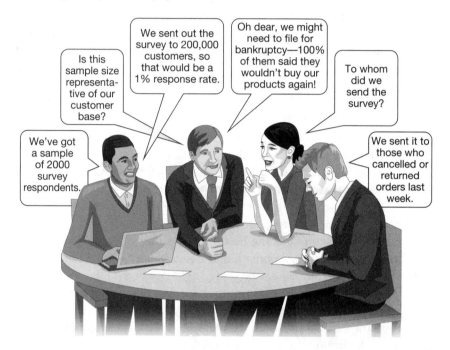

in fiscal year 2012. However, random sampling becomes more challenging if the population includes unknown elements. For example, it would be difficult to conduct a true random sample of all undocumented immigrants using primary care services in the Chicago metropolitan area. How would the researcher find these subjects and give them a number? While many statistical tests assume random sampling and random sampling is the most likely to produce a representative sample, it is not always feasible. Researchers employ four main types of random sampling.

Simple Random Sampling

A simple random sample is taken so that all subjects in a population have an equal probability of being selected (i.e., without any pattern). One way to obtain a simple random sample is to identify all subjects in the population by a number, then write each number on a piece of

Figure 2-2

How to use a random number table.

1765	4379	2763	205	162
9921	989	1908	7680	7554
3279	6589	442	5224	560
7995	8954	2603	8891	9452
5091	5276	1409	7835	9585
4904	2311	1572	2153	5850
8130	2667	9918	2402	6099
3916	2949	3512	4319	4669
7047	9501	8191	4008	8912
7643	3828	3091	541	2185
9027	7937	6953	6551	6476
2904	672	9849	7608	9079
1656	2693	2508	8439	5606
625	6222	3046	5476	2734
2127	6640	3880	2888	8009
3649	1356	3387	5712	8717
1843	8312	431	6023	9265
1170	6461	9818	6282	7340
799	578	3314	1014	6165
2718	4534	8512	2106	5639
9986	5254	8025	5435	1772
6853	3764	6210	1771	5364
5634	8882	2983	3709	8887
6272	1370	6786	6241	5413
9811	9361	4397	6349	3278
1810	6232	3288	749	6066
7109	4601	9517	9616	8715
6256	7868	7195	6087	1340
1625	8504	374	9999	7212
2240	9727	9955	1502	1748
7770	2716	549	6350	2521
7753	3475	5945	1812	6111

1. Pick **any** number as a starting point.

2. Assume that we are to take a sample of 10 from a population of 80. This means that we only need two digits to choose our sample. You can go any way you want from here, but I will go down to explain.

3. The first two digits, 89, is out of my range since I have only 80 people. The next two digits, 54, is in my range, so the 54th person is my first subject for the sample.

4. The next random number in the table is 5276, so we have 52 and 76. Both numbers are in range, so they will be selected for my sample. The steps continue until a sample size of 10 is obtained.

paper, place these in a hat, and randomly select the pieces of paper until the desired number of subjects for a sample is reached. A random number table or random number generator is also a useful tool for selecting a sample. **Figure 2-2** is an example of a random number table and shows a list of randomly generated numbers.

Systematic Random Sampling

A systematic random sample (**Figure 2-3**) begins with assigning a number to each subject in the population and then selecting every kth person (where k is the population size divided by the desired sample

Figure 2-3

Example of systematic sampling where every third subject is being selected.

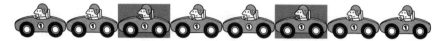

size). For example, if a researcher wanted to select a sample of 40 out of 800 subjects in the population, the researcher would select every 20th subject from the population since 800 ÷ 40 = 20. One thing to note here, however, is that the first subject will have to be randomly selected between 1 and 20. Systematic random sampling is a straightforward sampling procedure as long as the order of subjects is random. If the researcher is not careful about the order of subjects, it can create a nonrandom sample. For example, suppose that subjects were numbered in the repeating order of Caucasian, Hispanic, African American, and Asian. If a researcher begins with Hispanic as the first subject and selects every fourth subject, the sample would only contain Caucasian subjects except for the first person.

Stratified Random Sampling

To conduct a stratified random sample, divide the population into groups, called strata, based on important variables in the study and then randomly selecting subjects from each group. For example, suppose a clinical researcher is interested in learning how much stress men and women have about an upcoming surgery. The researcher will divide patients into two gender groups, men and women, and randomly select patients from each gender group.

A stratified random sample is *proportionate* if the subject size of each stratum in the sample is in proportion to that in population (**Figure 2-4**). In the above example, the sample is a proportionate stratified random sample if there are 60 men and 40 women in a selected sample taken from a population with 600 men and 400 women. Each stratum in the sample represents 10% of that in the population. For example, we could take a proportionate stratified random sample based on the geography of the United States in which 10% of residents in each region are sampled.

A stratified sample can also be *nonproportionate* if the subject size of each stratum in the sample is not proportionate to that of the population. For example, suppose that there are 600 men and 20 women

Figure 2-4

Example of proportionate stratified random sampling.

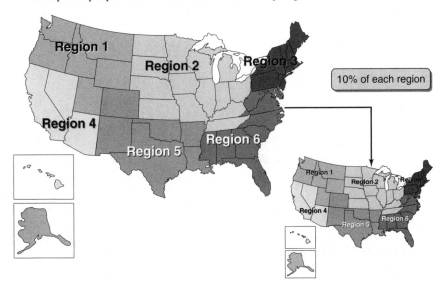

in a population. A proportionate stratified sampling will provide 60 men and only 2 women for a sample if a researcher were to select 10% in each stratum. However, this strategy would result in the group of women having too few subjects, causing the comparison between men and women to be meaningless. In this case, the researcher can select all 20 women and select 42 men, creating greater balance between groups.

In general, stratified random sampling is a more precise sampling procedure than simple random sampling. The accuracy of the sampling is maximized when subjects within a stratum are *homogenous*—when the subjects in the stratum are very alike. However, it can be a weaker sampling procedure when stratification is designed poorly and can be more complicated than the previous two sampling procedures.

Cluster Sampling

Cluster sampling is similar to stratified sampling. A cluster sample begins with dividing a population into different groups, called *clusters*. However, cluster sampling works better when subjects within a cluster are *heterogeneous* as much as possible (as opposed to stratified

Figure 2-5

Examples of cluster random sampling.

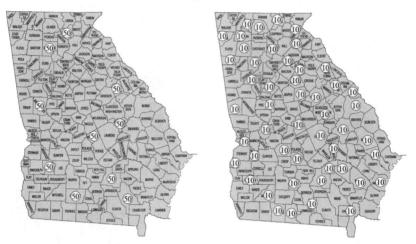

Random 10 counties
(50) people per county

Random 50 counties
(10) people per county

sampling, which favors homogeneous subjects). Cluster sampling is particularly useful when a population is large or when a study covers a large geographic area. For example, suppose that a researcher wants to do a study on health needs in counties in Georgia. It would be more efficient to randomly select counties and then randomly select subjects from those counties to study than to select subjects using simple random sampling (see **Figure 2-5**).

In general, cluster sampling provides less precision than simple random sampling or stratified sampling, but it is more cost-effective.

Nonrandom Sampling

Nonrandom sampling procedures do not rely on chance, and members of the population do not have an equal chance of selection. These procedures prioritize feasibility or access to the population of interest, and approaches other than random sampling are used to establish the representativeness of the sample. For example, if a researcher is testing an experimental drug for the treatment of pancreatic cancer, it will

EXTREMITIES:

SKIN:

GYN/G.U.:

Relevant Labs/Diagnostic Tests:

Social History

OTHER:

_____ Date: _____ Time: _____

be most important to find patients who have the disease, are willing to volunteer, and are candidates for an experimental treatment. The competent researcher takes care to collect data on the characteristics of each participant so that the representativeness of the sample may be ascertained at the end of the study. When employing nonrandom sampling approaches, the researcher trades statistical power for feasibility. Four commonly used nonrandom sampling procedures will be addressed here.

Convenience Sampling

Use of convenience sampling is based primarily on accessibility of subjects in the population. A popular example is using every student in a single course at a university, such as Psychology 101. In clinical research, convenience sampling is used extensively; nurses might be interested in sampling all pediatric patients hospitalized or all residents of a nursing home during a particular time. This sampling approach saves the researcher's time and effort more than any other methods discussed previously, but it will be less likely to represent the population.

Volunteer Sampling

A volunteer sample is taken in a way that only those who offer themselves as participants in the study are included as a sample (**Figure 2-6**). This sampling method is a relatively inexpensive way of ensuring a sufficient number of subjects for a sample. However, it tends to obtain skewed opinions on the characteristics of interests for a study, as this group of individuals will have a narrower range of opinions compared to a randomly selected group.

Quota Sampling

Quota sampling is done by dividing the population into mutually exclusive (not overlapping) groups and selecting subjects from each group, just like in stratified random sampling. However, in quota sampling, subjects within each stratum or group are not selected randomly. Rather, a researcher may take a sample within each group using convenience sampling. Quota sampling may also be a proportionate sample, but using convenience measures to select participants.

Figure 2-6

Example of volunteer sampling.

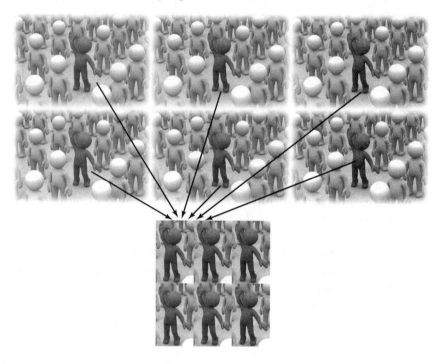

Snowball Sampling

A snowball sample uses word of mouth, nomination, or referral to accrue subjects. The researcher must make at least one contact with a subject, and then that first subject nominates or refers additional subjects based on personal contacts. Therefore, a sample will grow like a snowball rolling down a hill. This method is particularly useful for finding hidden subjects. For example, we might need to study teens who are injecting steroids. If we can find a few participants who are willing to ask others they know to participate, we are more likely to accrue a reasonably sized sample. The strength of this approach is in securing access to a sample of hard-to-find subjects. However, like all nonrandom samples, this method can produce a nonrepresentative sample of the population. In results, the statistics from this sample can be potentially misleading or biased if no other measures are used to improve the representativeness of the sample.

Nonrandom sampling procedures are generally easier and more cost-effective to implement than random sampling procedures. However, one should keep in mind that there is a greater chance that these sampling procedures will not produce the best representative sample. When a sample is not randomly selected, it is less likely to represent the population, and potential bias is introduced into the results. This potential bias is *selection bias*. If selection bias is not taken into account, it will reduce the accuracy with which the researcher can generalize results to the population. It is possible to estimate selection bias as a function of sampling error.

Sampling Distribution and Sampling Error

A **sampling distribution** is defined as a distribution of a statistic that is computed from samples. In other words, the sampling distribution of a mean or arithmetic average will be a collection of all means that we would compute from an infinite number of samples from a given population (**Figure 2-7**). Understanding sampling distributions is important because it is the basis of making statistical inferences from a sample to a population and helps us to look at how the value of a mean is like other possible sample means. For example, suppose a researcher selects 200 samples of 10 nurses from a large population and computes the mean of salary for each of the 200 samples. This will generate 200 mean salary measurements from each sample, and the distribution of those 200 mean salary measurements will comprise a sampling distribution of the sample means.

These 200 mean salary measurements will not exactly match the population mean (a parameter), μ, when they are selected randomly because each sample of 10 will have somewhat different nurses (**Figure 2-8**). This difference is called **sampling error** because the sample means will be different as the sample, a subset of the population, will not be the same as population.

Sampling error can affect our statistical estimate. When sampling error is small, it means that there is small variability in a sampling distribution and we can be more confident with the sample estimate. When sampling error is large, however, it means that there is a lot of

Figure 2-7

Sampling distribution.

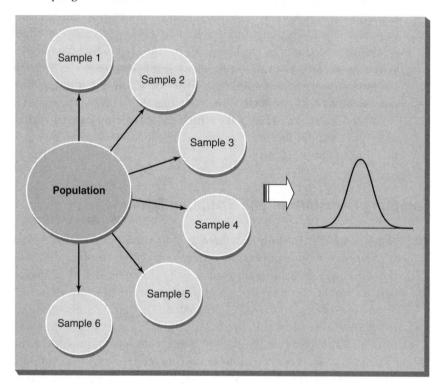

Figure 2-8

Sampling error.

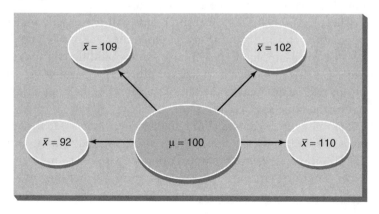

EVALUATING THE REPRESENTATIVENESS OF THE SAMPLE

- Is the choice of sampling approach likely to ensure good representation of the population?
- Has the researcher described the sample characteristics in enough detail so that the reader may evaluate whether inferences to the population are reasonably accurate?
- Is the sample size adequate for detecting statistical significance?
- Has the author identified limitations of the sampling approach?

---

variability in a sampling distribution and we will not be confident with the sample estimate.

There are two characteristics of the sampling distribution of sample means.

1. The mean of all sample means from a population will be the same as the population mean.
2. The standard deviation of all sample means (i.e., standard error) will always be smaller than the standard deviation of the population mean. It is computed by dividing population standard deviation by the square root of the sample size.

In research and evidence-based practice, the nurse needs to understand how representative the sample is and what strategies increase the likelihood that the sample statistics are an accurate reflection of population parameters. A critical analysis of the strength of the sampling approach and the representativeness of the sample helps us determine how strong the inferences from sample to population are.

Sample Size

Once we determine the sampling procedure, the next legitimate question is "How large of a sample size do I need?" If a researcher selects too few subjects for a sample, there will not be enough coverage of the population to make inferences. At the same time, too large of a sample may be costly and time consuming. So, how do we determine an adequate sample size? The answer to this question depends on many factors, such as the population size, the statistical procedure, and **confidence level** (this may be thought of as our tolerance for error). Most statistics books have a formula to calculate necessary sample size, and it is easy to find sample size calculators or software programs through Internet search engines. A popular procedure to calculate the necessary sample size is **power analysis**. This should be performed before a researcher begins the study to ensure that there are enough subjects in a sample to make appropriate inferences to the population. Power analysis will be discussed in more detail in Chapter 7.

Case Study

Hawkins, S. Y. (2010). Improving glycemic control in older adults using a videophone motivational diabetes self-management intervention. *Research and Theory for Nursing Practice: An International Journal, 24*(4), 217–232.

Older adults experience the greatest burden of diabetes. Resources must be available and accessible to empower older adults to perform diabetes self-care. The purpose of this study was to evaluate a videophone motivational interviewing (MI) diabetes self-management education (DSME) intervention to improve glycemic control of rural older adults. Sixty-six participants (mean age = 64.9 years, range 60–81) with uncontrolled diabetes were enrolled in a 6-month videophone intervention. Experimental group participants ($n = 34$) received weekly, then monthly, videophone MI DSME calls, whereas control participants ($n = 32$) received monthly videophone healthy-lifestyle education calls. Although both groups experienced a decreased HbA1c, there was a statistically significant difference in experimental group mean values ($p = .015$), but not in the control group ($p = .086$). The experimental group demonstrated statistically significant increases in diabetes knowledge ($p = .023$) and diabetes self-efficacy ($p = .002$). Experimental group participants with high self-efficacy in contrast to low self-efficacy had a statistically significant decrease in HbA1c ($p = .043$).

This abstract, published as part of a larger research report by Dr. Shelley Y. Hawkins, is a typical example of an experimental study on a topic of interest to nurses. Let us examine the abstract for key elements that help us understand the essential foundations of statistics and evidence-based practice.

Population: Rural older adults with diabetes

Sample: 66 adults between 60 and 81 years (note that the abstract does not indicate if this is a random or a nonrandom sample)

SUMMARY

There are many essential ideas to understand when learning statistics, and this chapter was intended to provide some of the most basic of these essentials. These include definitions and examples of descriptive and inferential statistics, the differences between population and sample, various sampling methods including random and nonrandom sampling approaches, and sampling distributions and sampling error.

Descriptive statistics communicate important elements of the collected data, while inferential statistics are used to infer conclusions from the sample to the population.

Populations are often too large and costly to use in research, so usually we take a representative sample of the population to conduct a study. The sample should be the best representation of the population possible so that we can make accurate inferences, and each sampling procedure has strengths and limitations. Random sampling methods are usually the strongest approach, but they may be more costly or not feasible, and they include simple random sampling, systematic sampling, stratified sampling, and cluster sampling. Nonrandom sampling methods are less likely to produce representative samples, but they are more expedient, less costly, and do not require the ability to access the whole population; they include convenience sampling, volunteer sampling, quota sampling, and snowball sampling. A researcher must consider the strengths and limitations of both random and nonrandom sampling approaches before designing a study.

Sample size is important as it can negatively affect our ability to make inferences if too few subjects are included or increase costs if too large a sample is used. The best sample size depends upon many factors, such as the population size, the statistical procedure, and confidence level.

The degree of sampling error helps us to understand how strong our inferences are from sample to population. The sampling distribution is one way of understanding sampling error.

The advanced practice nurse, nurse leader, and nurse administrator must be comfortable and skilled in the interpretation and application of the essential elements of descriptive and inferential statistics, sampling strategies, and evaluation of the representativeness of a sample in order to make sound practice decisions.

Critical Thinking Questions

1. What are the differences between population parameters and sample statistics?
2. What does the term *representative sample* mean?
3. Is it reasonable to say that stratified random sampling tends to produce a representative sample? Explain your answer.
4. In your daily life, find an example of the following:
   a. Descriptive statistics
   b. Inferential statistics
5. Why must the researcher begin with descriptive statistics when the goal is to conduct inferential statistics?
6. Use a random number generator or a random-number table provided in this textbook to generate 5 samples of 10 integers between 1 and 100. Are there any numbers appearing in more than one sample? What happens if you increase the number of integers drawn for each sample? Why do you think this happened? Explain in relation to standard error.
7. Suppose you are to conduct a study on patient satisfaction in a nursing home. Which sampling procedure will you utilize? Explain your answer.
8. Case study: From the following abstract, identify the population and probable sample type.

Case Study

Barkin, S. L., Gesell, S. B., Póe, E. K., & Ip, E. H. (2011). Changing overweight Latino preadolescent body mass index: The effect of the parent–child dyad. *Clinical Pediatrics*, *50*(1) 29–36.

Abstract

Background: Latino children are disproportionately burdened by obesity. *Objective:* To assess whether body mass index (BMI) change in preadolescents reflected that of their participating parent. *Methods:* A total of 72 Latino overweight/obese preadolescents (BMI $\geq$ 85%) and a parent participated in a randomized controlled trial. The intervention group received 5 monthly 60-minute sessions at a recreation center (group physical activity, goal setting). The control group received 2 standard-of-care clinic visits plus a group discussion. *Results:* Between baseline and 6-month follow-up, 47% of children (mean change $= -0.37$, SD $= 2.48$) and 63% of parents (mean change $= -0.88$, SD $= 3.53$) decreased their BMI. Parent–child dyad BMI change was significantly correlated ($r = .53$, $P = .001$). In linear modeling, those preadolescents in the control group were more likely to lose absolute BMI units (-0.96, $P = .03$); whereas those who had parents who gained BMI over the time interval were more likely to increase their BMI (0.17, $P = .008$). *Conclusions:* Obesity interventions should focus on the parent–child dyad.

Self-Quiz

1. True or false: Researchers take a sample from a population to infer the findings or results about a population.
2. True or false: Since descriptive statistics have a different objective from inferential statistics, they should not be performed together.

3. What is the general process of organizing, summarizing, and describing the collected data in an easier format?
   a. Inferential statistics
   b. Random sampling
   c. Descriptive statistics
   d. Hypothesis testing
4. A researcher would like to study average sodium intake across various racial and ethnic groups. However, he is concerned that sample sizes for some racial/ethnic groups might be too small to be useful in statistical analyses. What type of sampling procedure might be the most useful for his purpose?

REFERENCES

Baranzini, F., Diurni, M., Ceccon, F., Poloni, N., Cazzamalli, S., Costantini, C., . . . Callegari, C. (2009). Fall-related injuries in a nursing home setting: Is polypharmacy a risk factor? *BMC Health Services Research*, *9*, 228–237.

Barkin, S. L., Gesell, S. B., Póe, E. K., & Ip, E. H. (2011). Changing overweight Latino preadolescent body mass index: The effect of the parent–child dyad. *Clinical Pediatrics*, *50*(1), 29–36.

Buerhaus, I. P., Auerbach, D. I., & Staiger, D. O. (2009). The recent surge in nurse employment: Causes and implications. *Health Affair*, *28*(4), 657–668.

Seidel, S., Aigner, M., Ossege, M., Pernicka, E., Wildner, B., & Sycha, T. (2008). Antipsychotics for acute and chronic pain in adults. *Cochrane Database of Systematic Reviews*, *4*, doi: 10.1002/14651858

3

Statistical Essentials II: Measurement

Learning Objectives

From this point on, we will be building on earlier principles. In this chapter we will move on to statistical concepts related to measuring factors that are of interest to clinicians and researchers. Upon completing this chapter, you should be able to:

- Distinguish between independent and dependent variables
- Differentiate the levels of measurement and understand why this idea is important in statistics
- Discuss the application of levels of measurement to evidence-based practice
- Define reliability and validity and discuss the importance of addressing them prior to measuring variables with an instrument
- Understand how the quality of research is influenced by measurement decisions

Key Terms

Confounding variable	Data
Construct	Data set
Construct validity	Dependent variable
Content validity	Discrete variable
Continuous variable	External validity
Criterion-related validity	Independent variable

Instrument

Internal consistency

Internal validity

Interrater reliability

Levels of measurement

Qualitative variables

Quantitative variables

Reliability

Test–retest reliability

Tool

Validity

Variable

VARIABLES AND DATA

Researchers define variables and collect data to answer their research questions. By definition, a **variable** is a trait or characteristic that is assumed to vary, and **data** are the values of variables when they vary. For example, systolic blood pressure is a variable because it is a characteristic that we expect to change or fluctuate, both from one person to another and at different times within the same person (**Figure 3-1**).

Figure 3-1

Variables and data.

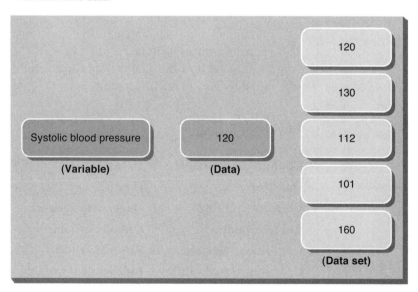

Each blood pressure measurement is a data value. A collection of these data values is a **data set**.

There are many different variable classifications. Variables may be *qualitative* or *quantitative*. **Qualitative variables** have values that are nonnumeric, while **quantitative variables** have values that are numeric. Systolic blood pressure may be seen as either qualitative—high, normal, or low—or quantitative—120 mmHg. In this book we will confine ourselves to numeric variables, as these are amenable to statistical analyses.

Numeric variables may be either discrete or continuous. **Discrete variables** have values that are countable but do not assume numeric value between countable categories. **Continuous variables** have every possible value on a continuum. Gender may be counted, as in there are 10 women in a waiting area, and is an example of a discrete variable; this is because, in the real world, there is no such thing as 10.5 women. On the other hand, systolic blood pressure ranging from 0 to 200 mmHg is an example of a continuous variable since we could measure the pressure anywhere between 0 mmHg and 200 mmHg. Conceivably we could measure systolic blood pressure to the nearest hundredth—120.05 mmHg.

Finally, a variable can be independent or dependent if a researcher is investigating the interaction between variables for statistical hypothesis testing. An **independent variable** is the variable that is either manipulated by the researcher or affects another variable. The **dependent variable** is the variable that is affected by an independent variable and becomes the outcome. For example, suppose a researcher is interested in investigating whether or not hepatitis B antigen affects liver function test results. The presence or absence of the hepatitis B antigen is the independent variable, as it affects the liver function test results, and the liver function test result is the dependent variable, as it is affected by hepatitis B antigen.

Consider another example. A researcher is interested in investigating the effectiveness of a newly developed medicine to treat constipation. The researcher devises an experiment in which the treatment group receives the new medication and the control group receives a placebo. The researcher measures the number of days between taking the drug and the first bowel movement among participants in both control and treatment groups. Here, the group assignment—treatment or control— is the independent variable since it is manipulated by the researcher and it affects the length of time until the first bowel movement. The number of days until the first bowel movement is the dependent variable, since it is affected by the group assignment or whether the participant received the new drug or the placebo.

With the previous two examples, it seems pretty clear how independent variables differ from dependent variables. However, students sometimes get confused about the number of independent variables in a study. Suppose a researcher is interested in investigating the licensure passing rates of graduating nurses from classes 2009, 2010, and 2011 at a public university. In this case, the graduating class is an independent or grouping variable and the passing rate is a dependent variable. However, students often think the three graduating classes are three *different* independent variables. Actually, graduating class is a single independent variable with three levels, since graduating classes are not different types of measurements (**Figure 3-2**).

Let us consider one more example of confusing independent and dependent variables. A researcher is interested in the relationship between social support and quality of life in older adults in assisted-living environments. The researcher hypothesizes that strong social support influences the quality of life of these older adults. In this example, it seems clear that social support is the independent variable and quality of life the dependent variable. However, the researcher could propose the equally valid hypothesis that quality of life influences social support; as such, we have

Figure 3-2

Types of variables.

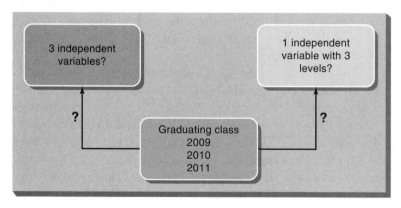

EVALUATING THE USE OF VARIABLES

- Has the researcher explicitly identified and defined the variables in the study?
- Is there a logical connection between the variables so that the reader can correctly identify independent and dependent variables?

flipped independent and dependent variables. In high-quality research, the researcher provides a logical argument for the choice of variables and the hypothesized relationship between them. The nurse using research for evidence-based practice must know how to evaluate such arguments and decide on the legitimacy of the approach used.

Understanding what variables are, how they are classified, and how they are related to one another is crucial in deciding which statistical method is appropriate for analyzing data. Practicing using statistics is an important part of becoming comfortable with evidence-based practice, and students will have to work with many examples to become proficient.

LEVELS OF MEASUREMENTS

After defining the variables of interest, the researcher must think about how to measure the variables. Data can take different forms depending upon how variables are measured. There are four common levels of measurement: nominal, ordinal, interval, and ratio (Table 3-1). It is important to understand the level of measurement because different levels of measurement require different statistical procedures. Measurement is also important for application of research to practice. For example, perhaps we are interested in implementing a wound healing intervention based on research evidence found in an article. The authors report that wounds healed 50% faster with the intervention than with another commonly used treatment. It will be essential to know how wound healing (the dependent variable) was measured to determine if the new intervention is an improvement over other approaches to treatment. Let us discuss each level of measurement one by one and see how they differ from each other.

Table	
3-1	**Examples of Different Levels of Measurements**

Nominal	Ordinal	Interval	Ratio
Gender	Places in a race (first, second, etc.)	Temperature	Age
Ethnicity	Age groups (18–25, 26–35, etc.)	IQ	Height
Zip code	Grade (A, B, C, D, and F)	SAT score	Weight
Religious affiliation	Histological opinion ($-/\pm/+/++/+++$)	Depression score	Blood pressure

In **nominal level of measurement**, data are classified into mutually exclusive categories where no ranking or ordering is imposed on categories. The word "nominal" simply means to name or categorize. Common examples in this level of measurement are gender and ethnicity; a researcher can classify the subjects as men or women (not both) for gender and as different ethnic groups (e.g., Caucasian, African American, Asian, or Hispanic), respectively. However, no ranking or ordering can be imposed on any of those categories as we cannot say one gender or ethnic group is superior/inferior, or is more or less than the other groups. Other examples of nominal level of measurement include religious affiliation (e.g., Christian, Catholic, or Buddhist), political party affiliation (e.g., Democrat, Independent, or Republican), and hair color (e.g., black, brown, or blond). Nominal measurement is often used in health-related research to characterize a wide variety of variables such as treatment results (improvement or recurrence) and signs and symptoms (present or not present).

In **ordinal level of measurement**, data are also classified into mutually exclusive categories. However, ranking or ordering is imposed on categories. A common example in this level of measurement is grouped age. People can be categorized into one of the following groups: (a) 18 and under, (b) 19–30, (c) 31–49, and (d) 50 and above. Here, we not only have distinctive categories with no overlapping (mutually exclusive categories), but there is a clear ranking or ordering among categories. Category (b) has older people than category (a), but younger people than categories (c) or (d). Other examples of ordinal level of measurement include letter grade (A, B, C, D, F), Likert type scales (strongly disagree, somewhat disagree, neutral, somewhat agree, strongly agree), ranking in a race (first, second, third, etc.), and histological ratings ($-$, $\pm$, $+$, $++$, $+++$). A common pain scale, ranking from 0–10, is a good example of ordinal level of measurement in health care, where 0 is equal to no pain and 10 is severe pain. What we cannot do with ordinal level of measurement is determine accurately what the distance between two categories is. We cannot say that the level of pain between 1 and 2 is exactly the same as between 3 and 4.

In **interval level of measurement**, data are classified into categories with rankings and are mutually exclusive as in ordinal level of measurement. In addition, specific meanings are applied to the distances *between* categories. These distances are assumed to be equal and can be measured. Temperature, for example, is measured on categories with equal distance, and any value is possible and can be measured; the distance between 35°F and 40°F is the same as the distance between 55°F and 60°F. However, in interval level of measurement there is no absolute value of "zero." Zero degrees Fahrenheit is not the same as zero degrees Celsius. Therefore, there is no absolute or unconditional meaning of zero. In addition, we cannot say 25°F is three times as cold as 75°F—that is, there is no concept of ratio, or equal proportion, in interval level of measurement. Other examples of interval level of measurement include standardized tests such as intelligence quotient or educational achievement tests. In health care we often use interval level of measurement for clinical purposes. Screening tests for depression, falls, or risk for pressure ulcers are examples of interval level of measurement.

In **ratio level of measurement**, all characteristics of interval level of measurements are present, there is a meaningful zero, and ratio or equal proportion is present. Therefore, it is possible to apply statistical tests with ratio level of measurement that are not possible with nominal, ordinal, or interval levels of measurement. For example, income is measured on scales with equal distance like temperature, but it also has a meaningful zero. The measurement of income for someone will be zero if they have no source of livelihood. We may also say that someone making $60,000 a year makes exactly twice as much as someone making $30,000 a year. Blood pressure is another example of ratio level of measurement, as it is possible to have a blood pressure of zero and a systolic pressure of 100 mmHg is twice that of 50 mmHg. Other examples of ratio level of measurement are age, height, and weight.

Level of measurement is important because it directs what statistical tests may be used to analyze the data sets collected by the researcher. Clinicians who understand the relationship between level of measurement and choice of statistical test are able to evaluate the strength of any given study. **Table 3-2** gives some examples of statistical tests per level of measurement.

Table 3-2	Statistical Tests According to Level of Measurement	
Independent Variable	**Dependent Variable**	**Statistical Test to be Utilized**
Nominal (control/patient)	Ratio (systolic blood pressure)	Independent sample *t*-test, paired sample *t*-test
Nominal or ordinal (low/middle/high systolic blood pressure)	Ratio (liver function)	One-way analysis of variance (ANOVA)
More than one nominal or ordinal (systolic blood pressure group + gender)	Ratio (liver function)	Factorial analysis of variance
Nominal (control/patient)	Nominal (nondiabetic/diabetic)	Chi-square test of association
Nominal + ratio (control/patient + age)	Nominal (nondiabetic/diabetic)	Logistic regression
Ratio (weight)	Ratio (systolic blood pressure)	Correlation, simple linear regression, multiple linear regression (if more than one independent variable)
Nominal with ratio to control (control/patient with age to control)	Ratio (systolic blood pressure)	Analysis of covariance (ANCOVA)
One or more nominal or ordinal (systolic blood pressure group)	More than one ratio (liver function + depression)	Multivariate analysis of variance (MANOVA)

There are times when a researcher may choose to reclassify or transform a variable's level of measurement. For example, blood pressure that is originally measured at the ratio level may be transformed to an ordinal level of measurement if a researcher categorizes the blood pressure in intervals of 40 (i.e., 0–40, 41–80, 81–120, and 121–140), or if transformed into categories of "high" and "low." There may be sound reasons for such transformations, such as wanting to make comparisons between people in those categories. However, transformation from a higher level of measurement to a lower level (ratio to ordinal, for example) limits analysis to those statistical tests for categorical measurements. Second, it will always result in the loss of information, as everyone with blood pressure between 41 and 80 is categorized into a single group. To return to our earlier discussion on variables, variables measured at the nominal and ordinal levels of measurements are discrete or categorical variables, and those variables measured at interval and ratio levels of measurements are continuous variables.

RELIABILITY AND VALIDITY

An important question in designing a study or evidence-based practice project is what measurement tools to use. A **tool** or **instrument** is a device for measuring variables. Examples include paper and pencil surveys or tests, scales for measuring weight, and an eye chart for estimating visual acuity. There may be one or more measurement tools available for variables of interest, or there may be none and a tool will need to be created. Whether you use an existing tool or you create one, you should make sure the measurement tool is the best approach for measuring the variable of interest. For example, suppose that you need to measure depression in older adults and you found an instrument, *Beck's Depression Inventory (BDI)* (Beck, Ward, Mendelson, Mock, & Erbaugh, 1961). Would you start measuring older adults' depression levels using the BDI right away? Probably not! First, you would want to make sure that the BDI is a good measurement tool to assess depression in older adults. The concepts of **reliability** and **validity** help us to make that decision.

Reliability

Reliability tells us whether or not a test can consistently measure a variable. If a patient scores 35 on the BDI over and over again, it means that BDI is reliable, since it is measuring depression consistently at different times. A researcher would not want to do a study with a measurement tool that is susceptible to the influence of factors other than the variable being measured.

There are three commonly used measures of reliability: internal consistency reliability, test–retest reliability, and interrater reliability. **Internal consistency** is used to measure whether items within a tool, such as a depression scale, measure the same thing (i.e., are they consistent?). Cronbach's alpha, the most commonly used coefficient, ranges from 0 to 1, with a higher coefficient indicating that the items are consistently measuring the same variable. **Test–retest reliability** is used to address the consistency of the measurement from one time to another. If the tool is reliable, the subjects' score should be similar at different times of measurement. Researchers commonly correlate measurements taken at different times to see if they are consistent, which is indicated by a higher coefficient. **Interrater reliability** is used to see whether different people's scores on a variable agree on ratings (i.e., are they giving consistent ratings?). Cohen's kappa is commonly used and ranges from 0 to 1, with a coefficient of 1 signifying a perfect agreement. For example, pressure ulcers are often scored on a scale reflecting depth, area, color, and drainage. If two nurses are using a rating scale to score the seriousness of pressure ulcers, we would want to know how consistent the scores are between the two nurses assessing the ulcers. Ideally, both nurses would score the same pressure ulcer very closely.

There are many factors that influence reliability of paper and pencil instruments, such as surveys or inventories like the BDI. The **first factor** is the length of the measurement tool. The shorter the measurement tool is, the less reliable it will be since it will be more difficult to present all aspects of the variable under study. The **second factor** is the level of expression of each item. If items are not clearly expressed, they will confuse people and it will be difficult to know whether the measurement is related to the variable under examination or to error. The **third factor** is the duration of time allowed for completing the measurement tool. If a researcher does not allow participants enough time, reliability will decline. The **fourth factor** is the condition of test takers on the measurement day. If a test taker is ill, tired, or distracted, these conditions can negatively affect the reliability of the measurement tool. The fifth factor is the difficulty of the measurement tool. If the tool is not designed at an appropriate level for the target audience, it can affect the reliability both positively and negatively; for example, the reliability will be too high if the tool was too easy for the target audience and be too low if the tool was too difficult for the target audience. Lastly, the researcher must consider the homogeneity of the subjects, that is, how similar the participants in a study are to one another. If the subjects in a group are homogeneous, one will expect a high reliability as people will produce similar scores. If the subjects in a group are not homogenous, one will expect a low reliability as people will produce a wide range of scores.

Reliability in its simplest form may be thought of as consistency or stability, and this is an important element to consider when choosing a measurement tool. However, consistency/reliability does not imply accuracy. For example, if we have a thermometer that consistently measures temperature two degrees above the actual temperature, it is a reliable thermometer, but clearly, accuracy is important as well.

Validity

Validity tells us whether or not a tool, an instrument, or a scale measures the variable that it is supposed to measure. There are three main types of validity: content validity, criterion-related validity, and construct validity. **Content validity** has to do with whether a measurement tool measures all aspects of the construct of interest. For example, the BDI will not be valid if it only measures psychological symptoms of depression and not physical depression symptoms. **Criterion-related validity** is how well a tool is related to a particular criterion. For example, suppose the BDI is determined to be an accurate measurement tool of depression. If you compare depression scores from another measurement tool for depression with those of the BDI and the score on the BDI is strongly associated with the score from the other depression measurement tool, then criterion-related validity is established. **Construct validity** is the extent to which scores of a measurement tool are correlated with a **construct** we wish to measure. A construct may be thought of as an idea or concept. For example, a researcher can ask himself/herself this question: "Am I really measuring depression with the BDI or could it also be measuring anxiety?"

EVALUATING MEASURES

- Are the measures congruent with variables identified in the study?
- Have the researchers reported on the reliability and validity of the measures and instruments?
- Have the researchers reported on limitations related to measurement?

Reliability and validity are two important concepts to consider whenever using a measurement tool. You should make sure either that the tool used is both reliable and valid or that its limitations are discussed if the tool is not proven to be reliable or valid. One thing to note is that reliability always precedes validity (Figure 3-3). An instrument can be reliable but not valid, but an instrument cannot be valid without being reliable. Unless you ensure that the tool has appropriate reliability and validity for your sample, you cannot make inferences following statistical tests.

Internal and External Validity

The quality of measurement in a study has a direct influence on the strength of the findings or inferences that we can make. Measures that are reliable and valid are more likely to produce accuracy in research

Figure 3-3

Reliability and validity.

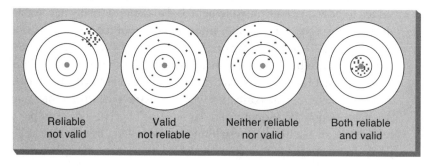

| Reliable not valid | Valid not reliable | Neither reliable nor valid | Both reliable and valid |

findings. This accuracy is referred to as internal and external validity. **Internal validity** is evaluated based on whether there is any uncontrolled or **confounding variable** that may influence the end results of a study. Such confounding variables may include outside events that happened during the study in addition to the variable under the study. These confounding events can actually cause a change in scores or measurement and result in less accurate findings. Changes in the participants due to aging or history may also introduce an element of inaccuracy. In longitudinal studies, for example, past experience with the measurement tool may also confound results, as merely having been exposed to the tool previously may influence the performance of the subjects on the later measurements. The choice of sampling, random or nonrandom, will also influence internal validity. Random sampling is designed to ensure that all participants are equal in every way, reducing the likelihood of confounding variables influencing the study results. Finally, human beings are prone to change their behavior when they know that they are being studied (i.e., Hawthorne effect) and this introduces bias that is difficult to quantify and to explain.

External validity is whether or not the results of a study can be generalized beyond the study itself. Can we make accurate inferences about the population from the sample we have selected? External validity is influenced by the quality of the sample. If the characteristics of the sample used in the study do not represent the population, the results from the study should not be generalized or inferred to the population. The second factor that influences our ability to make inferences is how well controlled the study is. Control over the independent variable is essential in experimental studies to ensure that the changes on the dependent variable are a result of manipulation of the independent variable only. Let us go back to our example of testing a new medication for constipation. We have asked participants to take either the new drug or a placebo and then measured the time from drug administration to bowel movement. However, what if we forgot to tell participants not to take any other laxatives while in the study? Now we cannot be sure if the time to bowel movement is related only to the new medication or if confounding variables such as the use of other laxatives resulted in the findings, and our certainty about the influence of the independent variable on the dependent variable is compromised.

Case Study

Seinelä, L., Sairanen, U., Laine, T., Kurl, S., Pettersson, T., & Happonen, P. (2009). Comparison of polyethylene glycol with and without electrolytes in the treatment of constipation in elderly institutionalized patients: A randomized, double-blind, parallel-group study. *Drugs & Aging, 26*(8), 703–713. doi: 10.2165/11316470-000000000-00000

In 2009, these authors published a study comparing the effectiveness of polyethylene glycol (PEG) with and without electrolytes for safely treating constipation. To ensure that the results of the study could be generalized to the target population and that the findings would be accurate, they used a randomized, double-blind, parallel-group study. Randomized means that the participants were randomly assigned to either the PEG with electrolytes or the PEG without electrolytes group. Double blind means that the participants did not know what group they were in, the people administering the PEG did now know which medication they were administering, and those collecting the data on effectiveness did not know what group each individual was assigned to. This study was designed with a high degree of control to ensure internal and external validity. The researchers found that PEG both with and without electrolytes were equally effective, but of course, the residents said it tasted terrible.

The researchers implemented two important approaches to ensure that confounding variables would not influence the dependent variable.

- Random assignment to ensure treatment and control groups are equal
- Double blind to reduce the Hawthorne effect

SUMMARY

This chapter is intended to introduce the essentials of measurement, including the definition of variables and data, different levels of measurement, reliability and validity of the measurements, and how these influence the quality of a study by promoting internal and external validity.

Variables are the characteristics or traits that are assumed to vary and data are the values of variables. There are four levels of data: nominal, ordinal, interval, and ratio. Nominal and ordinal data are both made up of categorical/discrete variables; however, only ordinal data has ranking or ordering between/among those categories. Interval and ratio data are both continuous variables with equal distance between intervals, but only ratio data have a meaningful zero and allow for proportionate understanding of the measure.

Reliability and validity may be thought of as the consistency and the accuracy of any given tool or instrument for measuring variables. Reliability and validity of measures influence the internal validity (accuracy of findings) and the external validity (ability to generalize from sample to population) of a study.

Critical Thinking Questions

1. What is the difference between the independent variable and the dependent variable? Give examples of each.
2. Imagine you are to conduct a study on how weight and age group (18–35, 36–53, and 54 and above) relate to systolic blood pressure. What are the variables in this study? Characterize each variable in terms of discrete vs. continuous, qualitative vs. quantitative, independent vs. dependent, and level of measurement.
3. Case study: From the following abstract, identify the population, probable sample type, independent and dependent variables, and level of measurement for each variable.

Case Study

Arslan, G. G., & Eşer, I. (2011). An examination of the effect of castor oil packs on constipation in the elderly. *Complementary Therapies in Clinical Practice, 17*(1), 58–62.

Abstract

This research, conducted at two rest homes in Manisa, Turkey, was undertaken to examine the effect of castor oil pack (COP) administrations on constipation in the elderly. Study participants were monitored for 7 days before, 3 days during, and 4 days after COP administration utilizing the Recall Bias and Visual Scale Analog (RB-VSAQ) as well as the Standard Diary developed by Pamuk et al. Eighty percent of study subjects had been constipated for 10 years or longer. COP administration did not have an effect on the number of bowel movements or amount of feces, but it decreased the feces consistency score, reduced straining during defecation, and improved the feeling of complete evacuation after a bowel movement, thus decreasing symptoms of constipation. We conclude that COP may be used for controlling symptoms of constipation.

Self-Quiz www

1. True or false? The length of a time in minutes a patient waits to be called at a hospital is interval level of measurement.
2. True or false? A researcher asks for a patient participant at a local hospital to rate the service as outstanding, good, fair, poor, and very poor. These data are measured on ordinal level of measurement.
3. Which of the following is the example of continuous variable?
   a. Zip code
   b. Gender
   c. Income
   d. Profit vs. nonprofit nursing home
4. True or false? An instrument can be valid without being reliable.

REFERENCES

Arslan, G. G., & Eşer, I. (2011). An examination of the effect of castor oil packs on constipation in the elderly. *Complementary Therapies in Clinical Practice, 17*(1), 58–62.

Beck, A. T., Ward, C. H., Mendelson, M., Mock, J., & Erbaugh, J. (1961). An inventory for measuring depression. *Archives of General Psychiatry, 4,* 561–571.

Seinelä, L., Sairanen, U., Laine, T., Kurl, S., Pettersson, T., & Happonen, P. (2009). Comparison of polyethylene glycol with and without electrolytes in the treatment of constipation in elderly institutionalized patients: A randomized, double-blind, parallel-group study. *Drugs & Aging, 26*(8), 703–713.

4 Working with IBM SPSS: Statistical Packages for the Social Sciences

Learning Objectives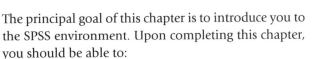

The principal goal of this chapter is to introduce you to the SPSS environment. Upon completing this chapter, you should be able to:

- Understand the application of pull-down menus
- Understand how to create a codebook
- Enter and import data into SPSS

Key Terms

Codebook

Data analysis menus

Data definition menus

Data file

Output file

Syntax file

Windows and general
    purpose menus

INTRODUCTION TO SPSS

You may be wondering why you need to be familiar with a statistical software package. We are certain that more and more nurses, especially those in advanced practice and leadership positions, will find that familiarity with software programs that facilitate quantitative data analysis will make their evidence-based practice work easier and more efficient. Let us take, for example, a chief nursing officer (CNO) of a large chain of long-term care facilities who must make decisions about staffing ratios and staffing mix to ensure that residents receive good quality care and to meet accrediting requirements. The CNO collects and enters data from each facility on daily resident census and absences among the nursing staff. Over time, the CNO, using the descriptive statistics that have been calculated, learns that peak absenteeism coincides with night shift duty and weekends (not a big surprise). Here, a software package can be helpful in calculating statistics as the volume of data can be large, and some necessary statistics can be very complex. Using these statistical findings, the CNO approaches the board of directors for approval of a significant increase in the night shift and weekend salary differential. Having well-organized statistics allows the CNO to advocate for policy changes to promote improved staffing ratios and avoid costly fees associated with violations of accrediting or inspecting bodies. Nurse managers, advanced practice nurses, quality improvement officers, and bedside nurses may all find occasions in which statistical results generated from data are required to make important policy and patient care decisions or influence those in a decision-making role.

The Statistical Package for the Social Sciences (SPSS) is one of the most popular statistical packages available. Statistical software packages are used to assist researchers and clinicians in answering practice and research questions. SPSS originated in the social sciences as the original acronym suggests, but it is utilized extensively in many fields because of its simplicity of use. This chapter will give you a brief overview of how to use this software package, and we will use SPSS outputs to explain various statistical techniques in later chapters.

Case Study

Hodgin, R. F., Chandra, A., & Weaver, C. (2010). Correlates to long-term-care nurse turnover: Survey results from the state of West Virginia. *Hospital Topics*, *88*(4), 91–97.

Researchers Hodgin, Chandra, and Weaver (2010) conducted a descriptive study that explored turnover with a convenience sample of 275 registered and licensed practical nurses employed in long-term care in West Virginia. They found that turnover was not associated with gender, educational preparation, job title, location, or facility size; instead, their findings indicated that turnover was associated with benefits such as pay, scheduling, and career ladder opportunities, and costs including travel time to work and facility characteristics.

The researchers in this case used a statistical test called the chi square test for independence in which associations between categorical/discrete variables are examined to make inferences from the sample to the population. They also used descriptive statistics to characterize the sample of professional nurses who participated in the study. All of these statistics may be accessed in SPSS.

Launching SPSS

You can either double-click the SPSS icon on your desktop, if available, or select SPSS from the Start menu (see **Figure 4-1**). Once you open SPSS, the opening screen should look like **Figure 4-2**.

Major File Types

There are three major file types in SPSS: data files, syntax files, and output files. **Data files** (*.sav) contain the actual data values. Data can be either directly entered into SPSS or be imported from other formats,

Figure 4-1

Opening SPSS from the Start menu.

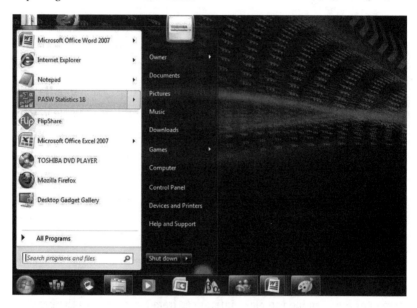

such as Excel, dBase, and Lotus files. Beginning with version 10.0, data files consist of two views, *data view* and *variable view*. Data view is where the data are inputted, and variable view is where the characteristics of

Figure 4-2

Opening screen of SPSS.

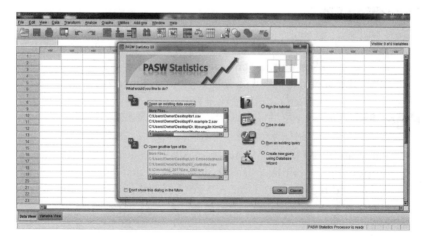

Figure 4-3

Different views in SPSS.

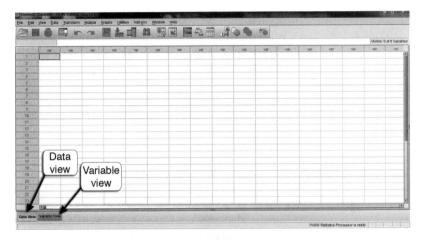

the variables, such as variable name, type, label, and values, are defined (See **Figure** 4-3).

Syntax files contain programmable SPSS commands to conduct analyses (as shown in **Figure** 4-4), and are a good alternative to using the interactive windows. Although there are certain analyses that can

Figure 4-4

Syntax file in SPSS.

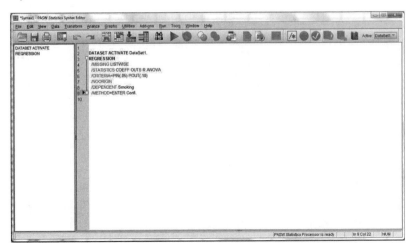

only be performed with syntax files, we will not discuss these in detail here, as most of the analyses for our purposes can be conducted with interactive windows.

Output files (*.spv) contain the results of the analyses as well as any error messages or warning messages (See **Figure 4-5**). An output file can be saved, edited, printed, or pasted into other applications such as Microsoft Word and PowerPoint.

Figure 4-5

Example output files in SPSS.

➡ Regression

```
[DataSet1] J:\Teaching_Spring11\NUR 489.01\Assignments\Assignment 1.sav
```

Variables Entered/Removed[b]

Model	Variables Entered	Variables Removed	Method
1	Self-Confidence[a]	.	Enter

a. All requested variables entered.
b. Dependent Variable: Smoking History

Model Summary

Model	R	R Square	Adjusted R Square	Std. Error of the Estimate
1	.856[a]	.733	.729	10.209

a. Predictors: (Constant), Self-Confidence

ANOVA[b]

Model		Sum of Squares	df	Mean Square	F	Sig.
1	Regression	16334.297	1	16334.297	156.737	.000[a]
	Residual	5940.246	57	104.215		
	Total	22274.542	58			

a. Predictors: (Constant), Self-Confidence
b. Dependent Variable: Smoking History

Coefficients[a]

Model		Unstandardized Coefficients		Standardized Coefficients	t	Sig.
		B	Std. Error	Beta		
1	(Constant)	93.887	5.782		16.238	.000
	Self-Confidence	−.972	.078	−.856	−12.519	.000

a. Dependent Variable: Smoking History

Types of Pull-Down Menus

As noted previously, SPSS is a relatively user-friendly statistical analytic software package due to the interactive windows. On SPSS 18.0, there are a total of 10 pull-down menus, which are categorized into windows and general purpose, data definition, and/or data analyses pull-down menus.

Windows and general purpose menus include FILE, EDIT, VIEW, UTILITIES, and HELP menus. The FILE and EDIT menus should be familiar to most of you as they are similar to those of other software packages. The FILE menu includes options to create new files, open existing files, or save and print the files or outputs. The EDIT menu allows you to find a case or variable, to cut and paste a data value, etc. The HELP menu includes an SPSS tutorial, which we recommend you use as needed as it provides detailed explanations on various topics for a new user. We remember the times when we first used SPSS, and we cannot even count how many times the HELP menu saved us! We hope you find this menu as useful as we do.

Data definition menus include DATA and TRANSFORM menus. The DATA menu includes procedures for inserting new variables or cases, sorting cases, merging files, splitting the file, selecting cases, and weighting cases. The TRANSFORM menu includes procedures for recoding variables, replacing missing values, computing new variables using existing variables, and a random number generator. These two menus become useful when a researcher wants to manipulate the file to resolve issues with violated assumptions or extremely unequal sample sizes for different groups. More on this will be discussed in Chapter 7.

Data analysis menus include ANALYZE and GRAPH menus. The ANALYZE menu includes both statistical and psychometric (reliability and validity testing) procedures, and the GRAPH menu includes various procedures for creating graphs and plots. One thing to note here is that some of these graph tools are available within statistical procedures under the ANALYZE menu. We will present how to use these functions to perform data analysis and create graphs as we discuss corresponding analytic procedures.

There are many icons on the menu bar that are associated with some of the same procedures as the pull-down menus. However, they will not be discussed as these icons display their function by placing the cursor over them.

Entering Data into SPSS

Completing a Variable View

When entering data into SPSS, the first step is to complete a variable view. This view displays the characteristics of the variables that must be defined so that the data may be entered appropriately into data view. These characteristics include variable name, type, width, decimal, label, values, missing, columns, align, measures, and role. Only the commonly defined characteristics are covered here.

The variable name should begin with a letter and only contain letters and numbers. It should not contain punctuation or spaces and cannot begin with a number. The name can be up to 64 characters in length, but we recommend using short names, approximately 8–10 characters, as variable names longer than this can create wordy outputs that may be difficult to read. For example, a question such, "How many times did you smoke during the past 3 months?" should be named "Smoke3" instead of using the entire question as a variable name.

Type includes many different formats, but *numeric* and *string* are the most commonly used ones. When the data are quantitative, such as age, the format should be left as the default, numeric. The format should be changed to string when the data are qualitative, such as responses to explain the choice of "other" categories in racial groups.

Decimal characterizes how many decimals are to be shown for variables. The default is set to 2, or the hundredths place, but unless data will be recorded or entered with decimals, we recommend changing to 0 to view the data more clearly.

Label is a description of what a variable represents in more detail. While we recommend using a short variable name, it may be easy to forget what the abbreviated variable name means. The label field allows up to 255 characters to describe the nature of the variable in more detail. For example, if we are entering data on wound characteristics, the variable name might be "depth," but the label may be much more detailed, such as "wound depth as measured in millimeters to the nearest whole number."

Values specify what numbers will be used to represent categories for categorical variables. You will need to indicate how numbers are assigned for categories, and this can be accomplished by clicking the gray square box with "..." on the right hand corner of a cell. Let us consider a case in which we are recording races. We assign a numerical value for each racial group: African American—1, Hispanic—2, Asian/Pacific Islander—3, and White—4. Values allow us to assign a number to a discrete/categorical variable.

Measures represent the level of measurement. Note that interval and ratio levels of measurement are combined in the term *Scale*. **Table** 4-1 shows the characteristics that define each variable, and we recommend spending some time using the pull-down menu to get the feel of it.

Table 4-1	Characteristics to Define in Variable View
Name	This will be the variable's name that will appear on the top row of data view. We recommend you keep the name to 8 characters or fewer, as a long variable name will not be shown nicely in data view. Note that you cannot include certain symbols, such as +, −, %, or &, nor use spaces.
Type	Define the types of the data. There are different data types such as numeric, comma, date, dollar, and strings; however, you will mostly use numeric (i.e., numbers for data values) or string (i.e., letters/words).
Width	SPSS, by default, sets this at 8 characters. You will be fine with 8 digits for a width of the variable most of the time, but it is subject to change to fit your needs.
Decimals	SPSS, by default, sets this at 2, or the hundredths place. You can change this to other values to fit your needs. For example, you can set it to 0 if your data value will be integers.
Label	Here you can describe the variable in more detail than you can in the short variable name. This will help you keep the variable name short but still remember what it represents.
Values	For categorical variables, you can assign numbers to represent different groups of people. For example, you can assign 1 for male and 2 for female.
Missing	You can assign numbers to missing data. Systematic missing, by default, puts a dot in the cell. You can also assign an impossible value for a certain variable to indicate missing data.
Columns	This is to indicate how many characters will appear in the column. You can change this to fit your needs.
Align	This sets where the data values in data view will appear.
Measure	This represents the level of measurement of a variable. You will choose either nominal, ordinal, or scale.

Preparing a Codebook

The next step of data entry is to prepare a **codebook**, which summarizes the characteristics of the defined variables. The codebook guides the creation of the data file and helps minimize errors with the data entry. There are other components that may appear on the codebook, but a typical codebook includes the following:

- Variable name
- Variable labels
- Values for categories of categorical variables
- Values for missing data
- Variable type (i.e., numeric or string)

Go to Analyze > Report > Codebook to create a codebook as shown in **Figure** 4-6. The variable view of the sample data set is shown in **Figure** 4-7. Creating a codebook as part of designing a study or evidence-based practice project is often a useful exercise for exposing flaws in measurement decisions or prompting questions about how data will be entered and analyzed.

Figure 4-6

Creating a codebook.

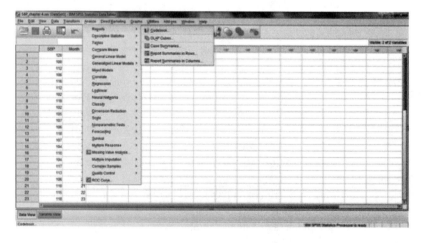

Figure 4-7

Variable view of the sample data set.

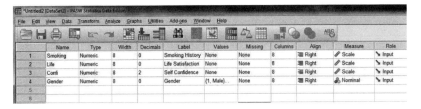

Entering Data

Entering data is simple after the first two steps are complete, as it will be just a matter of typing in the collected data values according to your specifications in the variable view. **Table** 4-2 contains example data for you to use to practice making a codebook and entering data. Once the prior procedures are completed, you should obtain a data set similar to the one shown in **Figure** 4-8. Note that Figure 4-8 is not in exactly the same format as you will see in SPSS.

Table	
4-2	**Example Data to Create a Codebook**

Smoking History	Life Satisfaction	Self-Confidence	Gender
4	40	86.30	1
27	80	70.18	1
5	80	61.52	2
10	67	55.51	2
9	58	70.10	1
13	48	95.52	2

Figure 4-8

Codebook of the sample data set.

Smoking

		Value
Standard Attributes	Position	1
	Label	Smoking History
	Type	Numeric
	Format	F8
	Measurement	Scale
	Role	Input
N	Valid	6
	Missing	0
Central Tendency and Dispersion	Mean	11.33
	Standard Deviation	8.359
	Percentile 25	5.00
	Percentile 50	9.50
	Percentile 75	13.00

Life

		Value
Standard Attributes	Position	2
	Label	Life Satisfaction
	Type	Numeric
	Format	F8
	Measurement	Scale
	Role	Input
N	Valid	6
	Missing	0
Central Tendency and Dispersion	Mean	62.17
	Standard Deviation	16.546
	Percentile 25	48.00
	Percentile 50	62.50
	Percentile 75	80.00

Confi

		Value
Standard Attributes	Position	3
	Label	Self-confidence
	Type	Numeric
	Format	F8.2
	Measurement	Scale
	Role	Input
N	Valid	6
	Missing	0
Central Tendency and Dispersion	Mean	73.1883
	Standard Deviation	15.08563
	Percentile 25	61.5200
	Percentile 50	70.1400
	Percentile 75	86.3000

Gender

		Value	Count	Percent
Standard Attributes	Position	4		
	Label	Gender		
	Type	Numeric		
	Format	F8		
	Measurement	Nominal		
	Role	Input		
Valid Values	1	Male	3	50.0%
	2	Female	3	50.0%

Importing Data into SPSS

You can also import data from other computer applications/software, such as Microsoft Word or Excel files. While there are other types of formats you can import into SPSS, only text and Excel files are discussed here as they are the most commonly imported files. Let us consider a situation in which your hospital admissions department keeps patient records using Microsoft Excel, a spreadsheet application used to collect, organize, and conduct arithmetic calculations. As a member of shared governance in the hospital, you have been asked to identify the top 10 admission diagnoses and the length of stay for each primary admission diagnosis. Excel data may be imported into SPSS to calculate a range of statistics that would help identify the most common diagnoses.

Importing a Text File

Text data are composed of contents directly inputted from the computer keyboard and can be easily imported to all computer software. **Figure** 4-9 shows the same example data we used in creating a codebook.

Figure 4-9

Text data file.

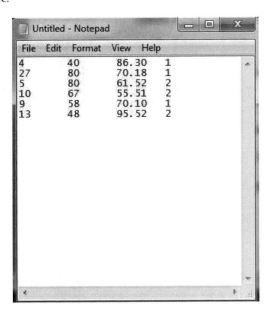

Figure 4-10

Locating and opening the desired file.

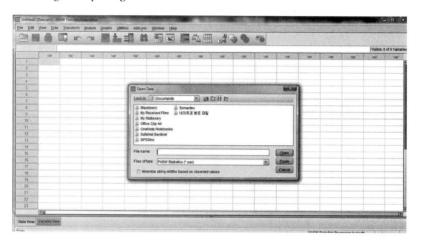

To import text, first, go to File > Open > Data. A new window (**Figure 4-10**) will appear. (**Figures 4-11 to 4-16** show the additional screens.) Change "Files of type" from *.sav to *.txt to show your desired text file. Click "Open."

Figure 4-11

Text import wizard step 1.

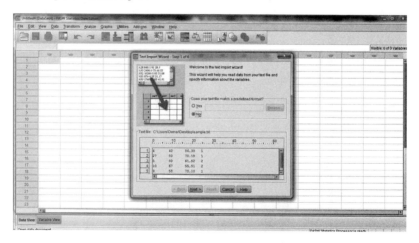

Without special changes, click "Next."

Figure 4-12

Text import wizard step 2.

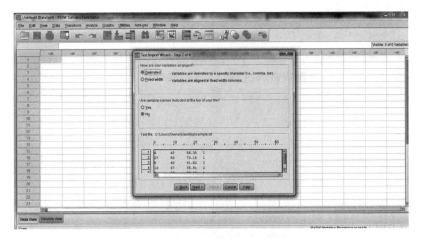

This text file contains the data values separated by tabs, so leave all options in default mode (i.e., delimited and "No" checked) and click "Next."

Figure 4-13

Text import wizard step 3.

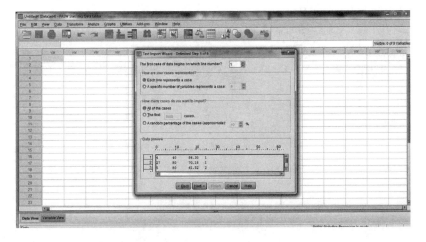

Our data display shows the first case on line number 1 and that each line represents a case. Because we want all of the cases to be imported, do not apply changes and click "Next."

Figure 4-14

Text import wizard step 4.

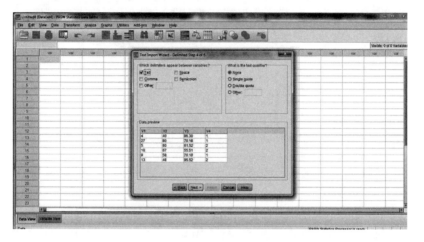

Our data values are separated by tab, so click "Next."

Figure 4-15

Text import wizard step 5.

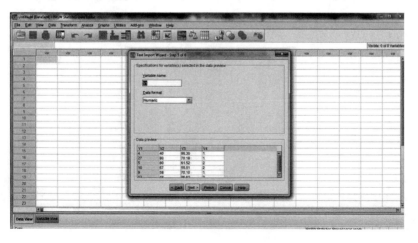

Here, you can specify the variable name and format by clicking each variable at the bottom of the window. Once you are done, click "Next" and then "Finish." You have now successfully imported a text file into SPSS.

Figure 4-16

End product of text import wizard.

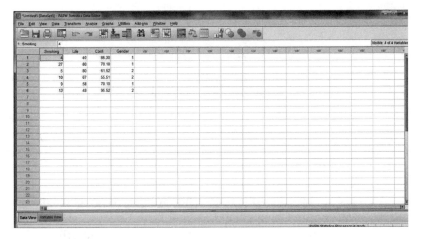

Importing an Excel File

Importing an Excel file into SPSS is easier than importing a text file. Assume the same data file was saved in Excel (**Figure** 4-17).

Figure 4-17

An Excel file.

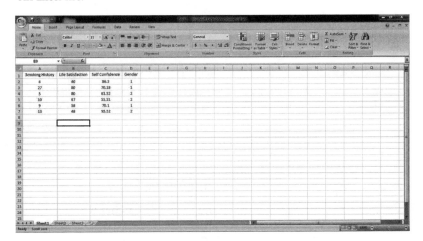

Figure 4-18

Opening an Excel file.

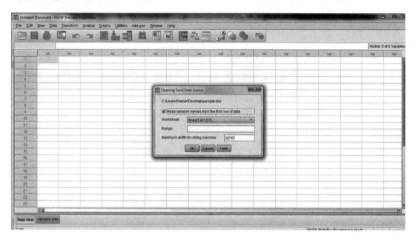

Again, go to File > Open > Data. A new window as presented in **Figure 4-18** will appear. Change "Files of type" from *.sav to *.xls or *.xlsx to show all Excel files. Open the file as we did with the text file.

Click "OK" with the default option if the first row of the Excel file represents the variable name. It should successfully import the Excel file into the SPSS software. You may change to variable view as needed.

There are many other functions that a researcher can utilize to help with data analysis, but we will discuss them as needed when we explain different types of statistical analyses.

SUMMARY

SPSS is a statistical software package that assists us in efficiently analyzing data to answer evidence-based practice and research questions, and it is one of the most widely used statistical software packages available.

There are three major file types in SPSS: data files, syntax files, and output files. Menus in SPSS are categorized into windows and general purpose, data definition, and/or data analyses pull-down menus.

Entering data begins with defining variables in variable view. Then, a researcher will create a codebook that provides information about the variables in a data set. This should help a researcher with data entry.

Data can be either directly entered into SPSS, or different types of data files can be imported into SPSS.

Critical Thinking Questions www

1. What does SPSS stand for?
2. Why is it a good idea to keep variable names short?
3. How will creating a codebook help a researcher in working with SPSS?

Self-Quiz www

1. True or false: SPSS only allows you to import the files in *.sav.
2. True or false: A variable name cannot be over 8 characters.

REFERENCE

Hodgin, R. F., Chandra, A., & Weaver, C. (2010). Correlates to long-term-care nurse turnover: Survey results from the state of West Virginia. *Hospital Topics*, *88*(4), 91–97.

Chapter

5 | Organizing and Displaying Data

Learning Objectives

The main goal of this chapter is to examine various ways of organizing and displaying data so that it may be understood thoroughly. Upon completing this chapter, you should be able to:

- Demonstrate techniques for showing data in graphical presentation formats
- Choose the best format to display the data
- Accurately interpret data presented on a graph or table

Key Terms

Bar chart

Boxplot

Frequency distribution

Histogram

Line chart

Percentile

Pie chart

Scatterplot

Stem and leaf plot

INTRODUCTION

Nurses in practice, administration, and research are often called on to present data in order to accomplish a variety of purposes—you may need to make a case for a change in practice or to promote the use of resources for a particular initiative, or perhaps you need to convince a patient that his behaviors are leading to poor health outcomes. After data collection is complete, what you have in front of you is a bunch of numbers and characters; it is important to be able to communicate the most salient aspects of the data to others. Similarly, as you are reading reports of research, you need to be able to determine if the researcher has made a defensible choice in the data analysis and presentation, as well as being able to understand a table or graph printed in the report.

If the number of data values is not large, it may be easy to interpret the data set. However, if the data set is large or complex, it could be very challenging to figure out what the data have to say. Imagine that you have two data sets: one with measurements on infant mortality from 20 countries, and one with measurements from 200 countries. Which one will be easier to understand?

So, how can the nurse represent data concisely, accurately, and clearly? One common approach is to present the data using tables, graphs, and charts. Depending upon the quality of our choices for display or the decisions of the researcher, data presentation can be clean and clear or muddy and misleading. In deciding what techniques to use for data display, we must ask ourselves two important questions. The first question is, "When should you use a graph or table?" Graphs and tables are likely to be useful when a researcher has a large amount of or complex information to report. If there are only one or two things to report, writing the findings in text may be just fine. However, as the volume or complexity of data increase, reporting in the text can become crowded and confusing.

The second question is, "What is the best type of graph or table to display our data?" Sometimes, a simple bar chart may be adequate to present data. In other cases, more complex displays may be needed to precisely communicate with the audience. Data displays should fit with the level of measurement and variable type and account for the audience characteristics.

Do you recall the different levels of measurement and types of variables we discussed in Chapter 3? Whether a variable is measured at the nominal, ordinal, interval, or ratio level will, in part, determine what presentation methods you will choose. Suppose the data collected are on the gender of subjects, so either male or female. Gender is measured on the nominal level of measurement. A simple bar chart or pie chart may be a good way to convey this information since there are only two response categories. Now consider a researcher who has collected the data on income of nurses. Income is measured at the ratio level of measurement and the data values are not limited within preset categories. A simple bar chart or pie chart will not be an appropriate display of these data because each income level reported by an individual subject will appear on the chart. Note that a bar or pie chart may be used if income measurements are categorized into a limited number of groups (e.g., 0–$25,000, $25,001–$50,000, and $50,000 and above).

As a nurse in an advanced practice, administration, or research role, you are expected to accurately interpret and decide on the best approach for displays of data. The goal of this chapter is to provide guidance on what factors to consider when choosing how to present your data. Commonly used graphs, charts, and tables are discussed. Remember, the mnemonic is KISA (keep it simple and accurate)!

Case Study

In 2010, the Centers for Disease Control and Prevention reported on sucides in national parks in the United States, noting that describing the scope and seriousness of the problem suggests that additional measures are needed for suicide prevention in the parks. The following line graph is a typical use of line graphing. The line graph is a useful way of displaying frequency of a set of values.

Number of suicides and attempted suicides in national parks, per year—National Park Service, United States, 2003–2009. *Source:* Data from Centers for Disease Control and Prevention (CDC). (2010). Suicides in national parks—United States, 2003–2009. *Morbidity & Mortality Weekly Report, 59*(47), 1546–1549. PMID: 21124294.

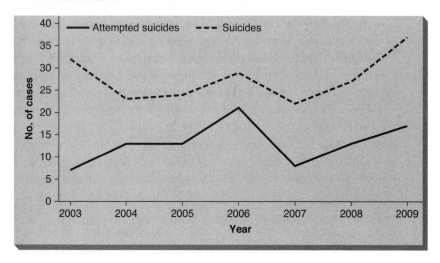

GROUPING DATA

One of the most common ways of presenting data is a **frequency distribution**, which shows a possible value of a variable along with the corresponding frequency of that value. The simplest frequency distribution has two columns, one for data values and the other for corresponding frequencies. **Table 5-1** shows an example frequency distribution of number of calls per night received at an emergency room in March.

The first column shows the number of calls received per night at an emergency room, ranging from zero to four calls. The second column shows how frequently an emergency room received the corresponding number of calls in March.

A frequency distribution table can be easily extended by adding additional columns such as cumulative frequency and cumulative percentage. Cumulative frequency is the sum of frequency of the current category with that of previous categories, and cumulative percentage is the ratio of cumulative frequency of the category of interest to the total

Table	
5-1	Frequency Distribution of Number of Calls at an Emergency Room

Number of Calls	Frequency
0	2
1	5
2	7
3	16
4	1

number of subjects. **Table** 5-2 shows the extended frequency distribution table of Table 5-1.

A frequency distribution can be either ungrouped or grouped. Our previous example was an ungrouped frequency distribution. If the data are measured at the categorical level, either nominal or ordinal, an ungrouped frequency distribution is the usual choice as there will be a limited number of category responses. **Table** 5-3 shows a frequency distribution table for gender.

If the data are continuous variables measured at the interval or ratio level of measurement, the choice of ungrouped or grouped frequency distribution depends on the range of the data values. If the range of data values is small, such as found in Tables 5-1 and 5-2, an ungrouped frequency distribution table may be still appropriate. If not, a grouped frequency distribution may be a more efficient way of displaying the data.

Table			
5-2	Extended Frequency Distribution of Number of Calls at an Emergency Room		

Number of Calls	Frequency	Cumulative Frequency	Cumulative Percentage
0	2	2	.06
1	5	7	.23
2	7	14	.45
3	16	30	.97
4	1	31	1.00

Table	
5-3	**Frequency Distribution Table for Gender**
Gender	**Frequency**
Male	20
Female	75
Total	95

Suppose that you want to create a frequency distribution of mortality rates of 200 countries. The data will range over many different values and an ungrouped frequency distribution table would have to be quite large to display the data. In this case, a grouped frequency distribution table will show the data more concisely as the distinct intervals of data values will be grouped to simplify the information about a variable. **Table 5-4** shows a grouped frequency distribution table of mortality rates of 200 countries.

A grouped frequency distribution table is a much easier way to convey information when the data set is large or complex, but there is a price you will have to pay. For example, how would you answer the question, "Which of these countries have an infant mortality rate of 5 or 6 deaths per 1,000 live births?" It is impossible to answer that question by looking at the grouped frequency distribution table. While a grouped frequency distribution provides good summative information on the data set, we lose information on individual data values.

Table	
5-4	**Grouped Frequency Distribution Table of Mortality Rates**
Mortality Rates (Death per 1,000 Live Births)	**Frequency**
0–10	2
11–20	5
21–30	7
31–40	16
41 and above	1

Figure 5-1

Selecting Frequencies in SPSS.

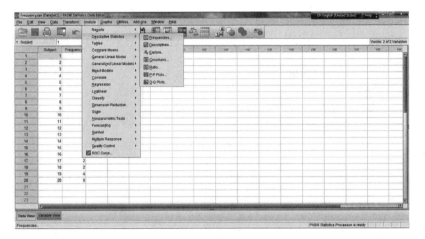

To create a frequency distribution in SPSS, you will go to Analyze > Descriptive Statistics > Frequencies as shown in **Figure** 5-1. In the Frequencies box, you will then move a variable of interest—in this case, Frequency—into "Variable(s)" as shown in **Figure** 5-2. Clicking "Continue" and then "OK" will then produce the output, shown in **Figure** 5-3.

Figure 5-2

Defining a variable frequency in SPSS.

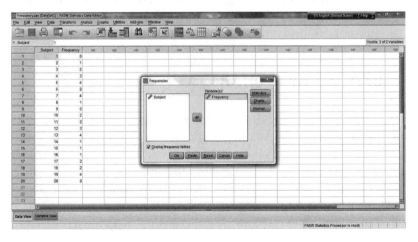

Figure 5-3

Example output of frequency distribution table in SPSS.

➡ Frequencies

```
[DataSet1] E:\2011\StatBook_2011\Chapters\chapter 5\Frequency.sav
```

Statistics

Frequency

N	Valid	20
	Missing	0

Frequency

		Frequency	Percent	Valid Percent	Cumulative Percent
Valid	0	3	15.0	15.0	15.0
	1	5	25.0	25.0	40.0
	2	6	30.0	30.0	70.0
	3	2	10.0	10.0	80.0
	4	4	20.0	20.0	100.0
	Total	20	100.0	100.0	

Which frequency distribution table is the best choice depends again on how the data are being measured and the range of values. If the range of data values is small, you would not want to create a grouped frequency distribution table and lose some of the information. If the range is large, however, a grouped frequency distribution table will convey information in a much simpler format even though some details of the information will be lost.

GRAPHS AND CHARTS

A nurse researcher, clinician, or executive may choose to convey information about data in graphs and charts that would be difficult or cumbersome to examine in text format. In fact, graphs and charts are the best method of describing the collected data when the data set is large. Graphs and charts are visually simple, so the data can be easily understood. There are many different types of graphs and charts available, but knowing the level at which each variable is measured will help you to determine what graphs and charts may be the best choice.

A useful chart or graph should show the data in a meaningful, clear, and efficient manner. Poor choices may lead to ambiguous or misleading interpretations of the data. Suppose a researcher is trying to find the best graphs and charts to present the collected measurements of weights of 100 patients. Since each patient will have different measurements in weight, choosing a pie chart as a description method will not display the data clearly, as shown in **Figure** 5-4. When there are many

Figure 5-4

Mistakenly used pie chart.

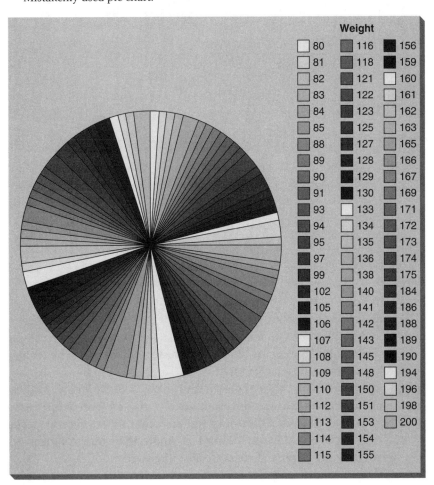

Figure 5-5

Histogram using the same data set as Figure 5-3.

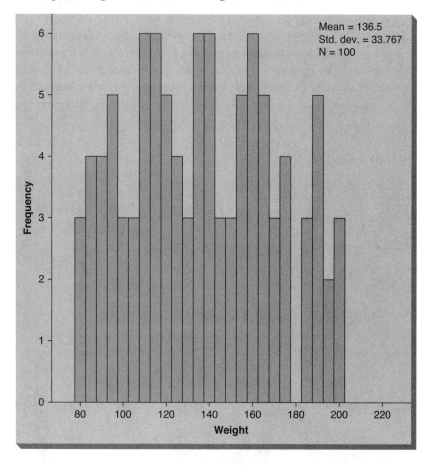

data values to display, seeing each data value as a separate category does not help us in understanding the data very clearly, efficiently, or meaningfully. In this case, the use of a histogram is a much better way to understand the data (**Figure 5-5**).

There are many types of graphs and charts in SPSS, and we will explain how to create each with examples of variables. Each data set used here is also included in the online resources for this text, accessed using the code found in the front of this text. Appropriate levels of measurement for each graph and chart are also discussed.

Discrete or Categorical Data

Bar charts and pie charts are two useful ways to represent discrete data (i.e., data that are categorical with fixed number of categories measured at the nominal or ordinal level). They are commonly used charts as they are easy to create, use, and interpret.

Bar Chart

The **bar chart** is the most appropriate choice for variables measured at the nominal and ordinal level of measurement and can be used to display one or more variables. If a bar chart is used with the ordinal level of measurement, ordering the rank helps the reader in interpreting the chart (e.g., if discussing pressure ulcers, listing the measurements in order—Stage I, Stage II, Stage III, Stage VI). A typical bar chart has the response categories on the horizontal axis and the frequencies of each category on the vertical axis; this helps you discern much about the data, such as the most/least common category, the difference of one bar relative to the other, and changes in frequency over time.

To create almost any chart or graph for a variable in SPSS, you will go to Graph > Legacy Dialogues and select the type of graph/chart desired—in this case, Bar, as shown in **Figure 5-6**. In the Bar Charts box,

Figure 5-6

Selecting a bar chart in SPSS.

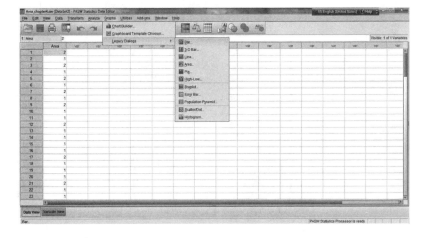

Figure 5-7

Selecting a simple bar chart in SPSS.

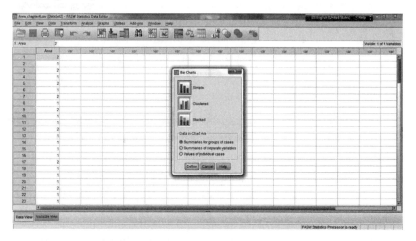

you will leave "Simple" and "Summaries for groups of cases" selected as default, and click "Define" as shown in **Figure 5-7**. In the Define Simple Bar box, you will then move the variable of interest—in this example, Location—into "Category Axis" as shown in **Figure 5-8**. Click "OK" to produce the output (**Figure 5-9**).

Figure 5-8

Defining a variable in a bar chart in SPSS.

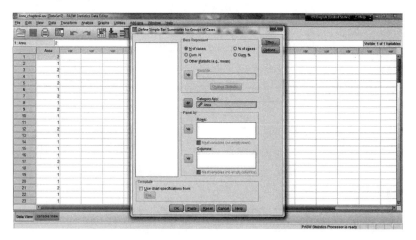

Figure 5-9

Example bar chart for nurses' job location.

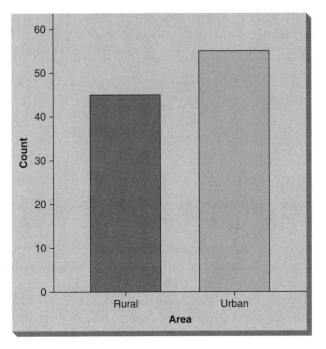

Bar charts can be created both vertically and horizontally. Additional examples where a bar chart can be handy to present the data include ethnicity, eye color, current position of nurses (staff nurse, administrative nurse, and dean of nursing), and gender.

Pie Chart

A **pie chart** is a circular chart where pieces within the chart represent a corresponding proportion of each category, and it is an appropriate choice for nominal and ordinal level of measurement. A pie chart is simple to create, use, and understand, much like a bar chart when it is created for a single variable. You can tell much about the data, such as the most commonly occurring class of the whole and relative size of different classes. However, it may be difficult to compare data across different pie charts.

Figure 5-10

Selecting a pie chart in SPSS.

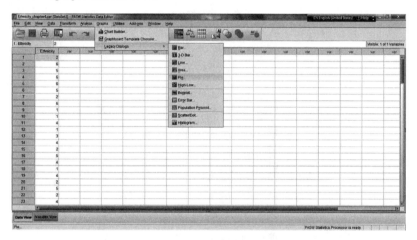

To create a simple pie chart for a variable in SPSS, you will go to Graph > Legacy Dialogues > Pie, as shown in **Figure 5-10**. In the Pie Charts box, you will leave "Summaries for groups of cases" checked as default and click "Define" as shown in **Figure 5-11**. In Define slices, you will then move a variable of interest, Ethnicity, into "Define Slices by" as shown in **Figure 5-12**. Clicking "OK" will then produce the output. Example output is shown in **Figure 5-13**.

Figure 5-11

Selecting a simple pie chart in SPSS.

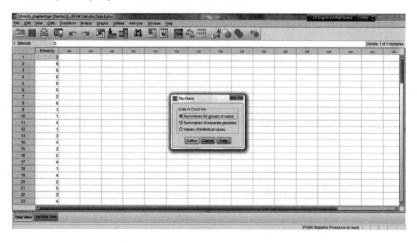

Figure 5-12

Defining a variable in a pie chart in SPSS.

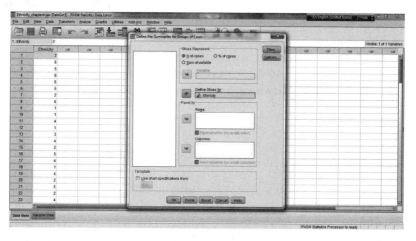

Figure 5-13

Example pie chart.

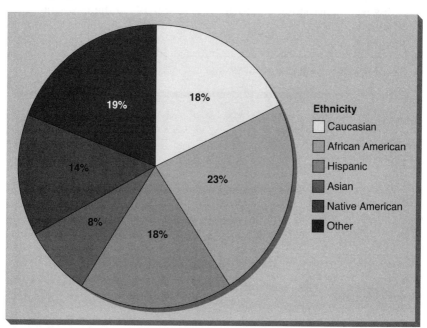

Continuous Data

When the variable is measured on continuous levels of measurement (i.e., interval and ratio), both bar charts and pie charts become inefficient in displaying the collected data. It is important to show how the data are distributed with continuous data, since the data values can range differently, unlike with categorical data. Better choices for continuous variables are histograms, stem and leaf plots, and box plots.

Histogram

A **histogram** is similar to a bar chart in structure, which explains why histograms are often mistaken for bar charts. However, you can think of it as a graphical way of presenting information from a frequency distribution. It organizes a group of data points into a number of intervals, and the bar in a histogram represents the frequency in corresponding intervals, not in predefined limited numbers of categories as with a bar chart. You can tell much about the data, such as general shape of the data distribution (i.e., which way most data values are leaning towards) and the most commonly occurring data value.

To create a histogram in SPSS, you will go to Graph > Legacy Dialogues > Histogram as shown in **Figure** 5-14. In the Histogram box,

Figure 5-14

Selecting a histogram chart in SPSS.

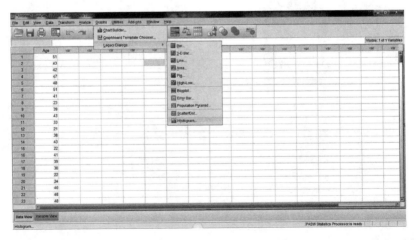

Figure 5-15

Defining a variable in a histogram in SPSS.

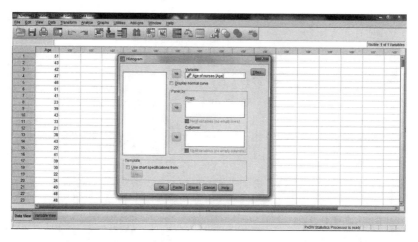

you will then move a variable of interest, Age, into "Variable" as shown in **Figure 5-15**. Clicking "OK" will then produce the output. Example output is shown in **Figure 5-16**. Note that a histogram can be obtained in other places, such as "Explore."

Stem and Leaf Plot

Stem and leaf plots are also good charts for showing the distribution of the continuous data. They are similar to a histogram, but have greater flexibility to show more information. While a histogram only shows the overall shape of distribution, a **stem and leaf plot** also shows information regarding individual data values. To create a stem and leaf plot in SPSS, you will go to Analyze > Descriptive Statistics > Explore as shown in **Figure 5-17**. In the Explore box, you will move a variable of interest, Job Satisfaction, into "Dependent List" as shown in **Figure 5-18**. Note that you can move the categorical variable into "Factor List" if you want to create separate stem and leaf plots for a categorical variable; this will create separate plots for different categories of the variable. Stem and leaf plot is checked as the default in "Plots" button, so clicking "OK" will then produce the output. **Figure 5-19** is an example of a stem and leaf plot.

Figure 5-16

Example histogram.

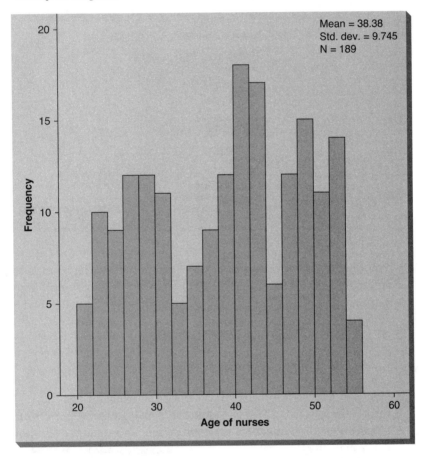

As you can see in Figure 5-19, the variable, Satisfaction, looks similar on both sides from the center and the actual data values are shown. In this way, stem and leaf plots not only show the distribution, but also information about individual data values.

Boxplot

A **boxplot** can be used to display more information than any other chart discussed so far in this chapter. It is a good choice for variables measured

Figure 5-17

Selecting a stem and leaf plot in SPSS.

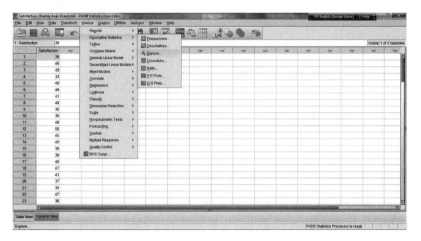

on the continuous scale and allows for comparisons across groups. A boxplot does not show individual data values like a stem and leaf plot, but it does display other information, such as the overall distribution, the center of the distribution, the quartile, and any possible outliers.

Figure 5-18

Defining a variable in a stem and leaf plot in SPSS.

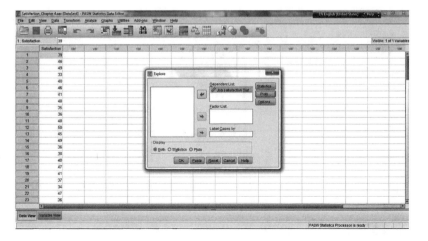

Figure 5-19

Example stem and leaf plot.

```
Job satisfaction Stem-and-Leaf Plot

Frequency         Stem &   Leaf

     4.00           3 .  0111
    15.00           3 .  222222222233333
     5.00           3 .  44455
    15.00           3 .  666666666667777
     9.00           3 .  888999999
    18.00           4 .  000000011111111111
     6.00           4 .  223333
     7.00           4 .  4445555
     8.00           4 .  66777777
    10.00           4 .  8888999999
     3.00           5 .  000

 Stem width:            10
 Each leaf:             1 case(s)
```

To create a boxplot in SPSS, you will go to Graph > Legacy Dialogues > Boxplot as shown in **Figure** 5-20. In the Boxplot box, you will leave "Simple" and "Summaries for groups of cases" selected as

Figure 5-20

Selecting Boxplot in SPSS.

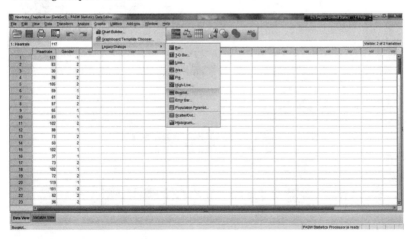

Figure 5-21

Selecting a simple boxplot in SPSS.

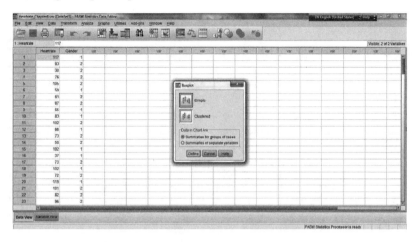

default, and click "Define" as shown in **Figure 5-21**. In the Define Simple Boxplot box, you will move a variable of interest, Job satisfaction, into "Variable" and Gender into "Category Axis" as shown in **Figure 5-22**. Clicking "OK" will then produce the output. An example output is shown in **Figure 5-23**.

Figure 5-22

Defining variables in a boxplot in SPSS.

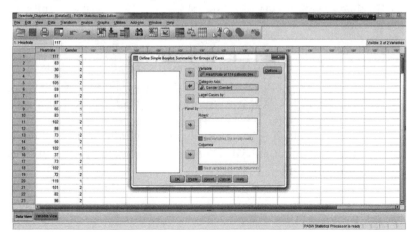

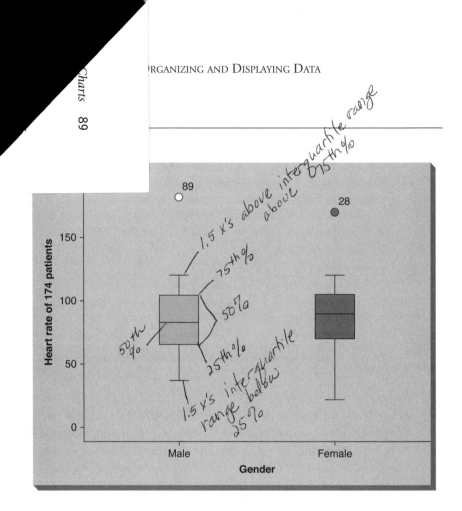

A boxplot can be drawn both vertically, as shown in Figure 5-23, and horizontally. It is one of the important charts used to describe the data in exploratory data analysis. Interpretation of a boxplot is as follows.

- The box in the plot contains the middle 50% of the data set. The middle line in the box represents the 50th percentile, the exact middle number of the entire data set, while the upper edge represents the 75th percentile and the lower edge represents the 25th percentile.
- If the middle line is not exactly in the middle of the box, it is an indication that the data is not equally distributed in both sides from the center.
- The ends of the vertical lines, which are called "whiskers," represent the minimum and maximum data values. The lower

whisker equals 1.5 times the interquartile range (IQR) below the first quartile (25th percentile), and the upper whisker equals 1.5 times the IQR above the third quartile (75th percentile).

- Any data value outside of the whiskers is considered to be a possible outlier, which is defined as an unusual data value in the current data set.

We need to give you an explanation on percentile before we finish a discussion on a boxplot. **Percentile** is a measure of location and tells us how many data values fall below a certain percentage of observations. For example, it means that you did better than 75% of your class on a certain exam if you have obtained the 75th percentile.

OTHER GRAPHS AND CHARTS

There are other graphs and charts that may be useful to display data. They include line chart and scatter plot. Both of them can be used to examine variables over time or against each other. The following will clearly illustrate the distinction between the two.

Line Chart

Like the bar chart and pie chart, the **line chart** is another good choice for displaying the frequency of categories. It is created by connecting dots, representing the data values of each category as shown in **Figure 5-24**. In this example, the horizontal axis represents "Month," a categorical variable, and the vertical axis represents "Systolic Blood Pressure," a continuous variable.

A line chart is useful when trying to find and compare changes over time or when trying to define meaningful patterns of variables. To create a line chart in SPSS, you will go to Graph > Legacy Dialogues > Line as shown in **Figure 5-25**. In the Line Charts box, you will leave "Simple" and "Summaries for groups of cases" selected as default, and click "Define" as shown in **Figure 5-26**. In the Define Simple Line box, you will then move a variable of interest, Systolic Blood Pressure, into "Variable" after clicking a radio button for "Other statistics" (e.g., mean) and Month into "Category Axis" as shown in **Figure 5-27**.

Figure 5-24

Example line chart.

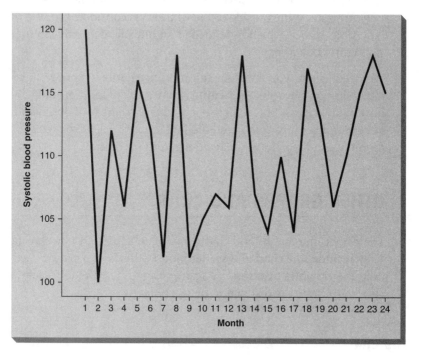

Figure 5-25

Selecting a line chart window in SPSS.

Figure 5-26

Selecting a simple line chart window in SPSS.

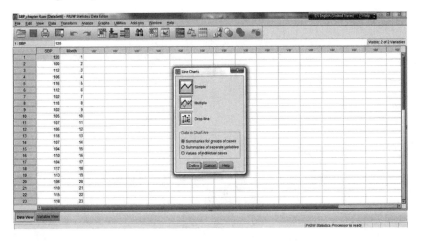

Figure 5-27

Defining a variable in a line chart in SPSS.

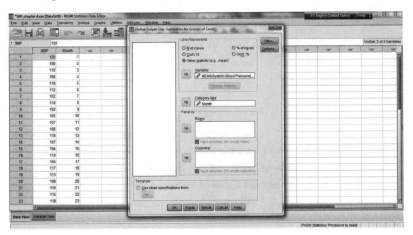

Scatterplot

Scatterplots are used when a researcher wishes to examine the relationship between two continuous variables—for example, age and systolic blood pressure. Relationships can be in either positive or

Figure 5-28

Example scatterplot.

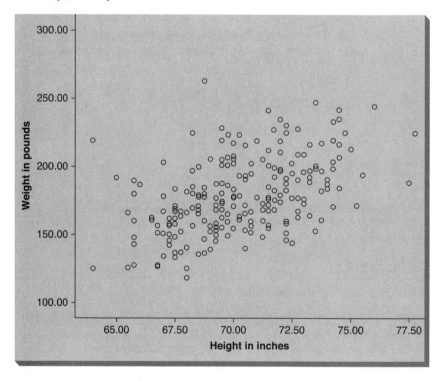

negative directions. A positive relationship means that both variables move in the same direction, such as increased smoking and the increased probability of getting lung cancer, while a negative relationship means that the variables move in opposite directions, such as high self-esteem and increased depression. **Figure** 5-28 shows an example of a scatter plot.

To create a scatterplot in SPSS, you will go to Graph > Legacy Dialogues > Scatter/Dot as shown in **Figure 5-29**. In the Scatter/Dot box, you will leave "Simple Scatter" selected as default, and click "Define" as shown in **Figure 5-30**. In the Simple Scatterplot box, you will move an independent variable, Height, into "X Axis" and a dependent variable, Weight, into "Y Axis" as shown in **Figure 5-31**. Clicking "OK" will then produce the output.

Figure 5-29

Selecting a scatterplot in SPSS.

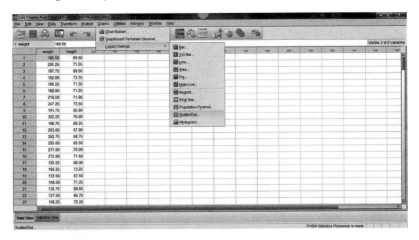

PRESENTING THE DATA IN THE BEST FORMAT

We have discussed many different methods of displaying the collected data, and most of these charts are easy to create, use, and understand. However, if any of these charts is not carefully designed to eliminate

Figure 5-30

Selecting a simple scatterplot in SPSS.

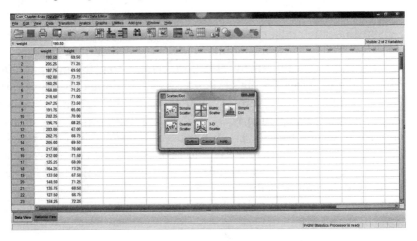

Figure 5-31

Defining variables in a scatterplot in SPSS.

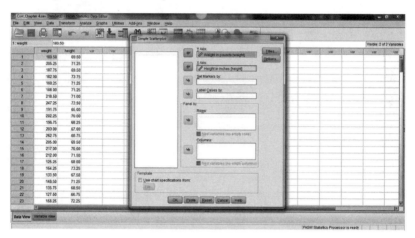

possible sources of bad graphical display, they can present false information. In ensuring the use of the best type of graph for your data, there are some things you should consider when you display your data in graphs or charts.

First, you need to ask yourself whether you have chosen the most appropriate type of graph for the data. For example, you would not want to generate a histogram to display the data values on an ethnicity variable or a bar chart for sodium content level of 100 patients. Or, you may ask yourself whether a bar chart or pie chart will display frequencies on different diet types better. Second, you should make sure that you have provided enough information on each component of the graph. The title should be clearly stated and the variable(s) should be clearly named. Third, make sure that the independent variable is placed on the horizontal axis while the dependent variable is placed on the vertical axis. Reversed, the graph may illustrate a different picture than what you want to show. Finally, you also have to ensure that the graph has been drawn on the proper scale, as it may show a different scenario than what it actually is occurring if it is incorrectly drawn. **Figure 5-32** is a perfect example of how an inappropriately scaled graph can be misleading. While the data do not show a strong relationship between number of years worked at

Figure 5-32

Example of data distortion.

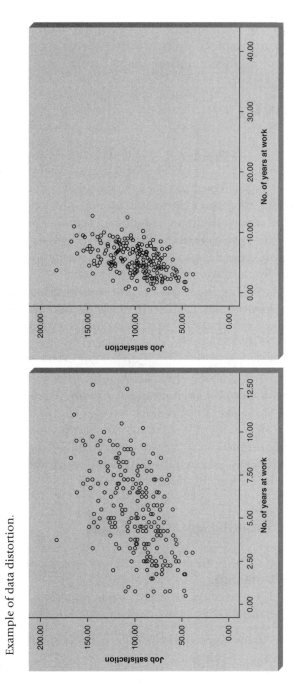

the current job and job satisfaction (as shown in the graph on the left), the graph on the right shows a very strong positive relationship due to the inappropriately defined scale.

SUMMARY

Graphs and charts are a useful and efficient way of displaying data. When the table, graph, or plot is created carefully and appropriately, your data will be more clearly understood and more meaningful. The careful nurse researcher, clinician, and administrator should keep in mind what each chart is good for and choose a chart accordingly.

Bar charts and pie charts are good for displaying the frequency or percentage of given categories. Line charts are also good when the variable for the horizontal axis is categorical.

Histograms, stem and leaf plots, and boxplots are good for displaying the distribution of continuously measured variables. A histogram is similar to a bar chart in structure, but it is used to show the distribution of data values in a user-defined range. Stem and leaf plots show the same information as a histogram, but they show the actual data. A boxplot is probably the chart with the most information, as it shows information on minimum and maximum values, the center values, and the 25th and 75th percentiles.

However, all of these charts can be easily manipulated to produce false information if they are not carefully designed. Therefore, a researcher should carefully think about which type of graphs or charts will be the best for the collected data.

Critical Thinking Questions www.

1. What is the purpose of constructing a graph or table to display information about a variable?
2. Levels of measurement are an important factor in determining which chart to use. Explain why this is the case.

Refer to the graph on the next page for questions 3–5.

3. Does this chart seem to be appropriate for this data? Why or why not? Explain your answer.

4. Is the title appropriately worded?
5. Is there any component of this chart that you think it is not adequately done? Explain.

Self-Quiz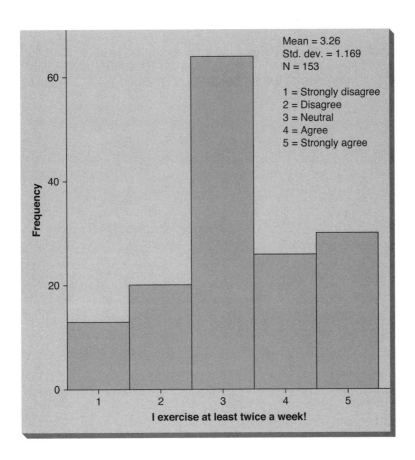

1. True or false: A histogram is useful when a researcher is trying to display information about a categorical variable.
2. True or false: Bar charts and pie charts can convey similar types of information.
3. True or false: There is no such chart that allows a researcher to identify possible outliers.

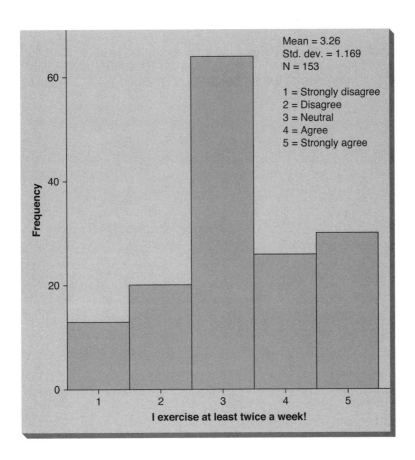

4. Which of the following is a good example of data that can be appropriately displayed with a line chart?
   a. Ethnicity
   b. Systolic blood pressure
   c. Income
   d. Age
5. Which of these charts allows a researcher to examine a possible relationship between two continuous variables?
   a. Histogram
   b. Bar chart
   c. Scatterplot
   d. Line chart

REFERENCE

Centers for Disease Control and Prevention (CDC). (2010). Suicides in national parks—United States, 2003–2009. *Morbidity & Mortality Weekly Report, 59*(47), 1546–1549. PMID: 21124294.

Chapter

6

Descriptive Statistics

Learning Objectives

The principal goal of this chapter is to explain what descriptive statistics are and how they can be used to examine a normal distribution. Confidence intervals are also discussed. This chapter will prepare you to:

- Explain the purpose of descriptive statistics
- Compute measures of central tendency
- Compute measures of variability
- Understand and choose the best central tendency and variability statistic for different levels of measurement
- Describe the normal distribution and associated statistics and probabilities
- Apply concepts of interval estimates and describe methods for determining sample size
- Apply understanding of central tendency and variability to nursing practice

Key Terms

Bimodal distribution
Central tendency
Confidence interval
Degrees of freedom (df)
Descriptive statistics
Interquartile range
Mean

Median
Mode
Multimodal distribution
Normal distribution
Point estimates
Range
Skewness/kurtosis

Standard deviation	Variance
Standard normal distribution	Variation
Unimodal distribution	Z-scores/standardized scores
Variability	

INTRODUCTION

We have seen how nurses in practice can present data in a variety of formats such as graphs, charts, and tables. These graphical formats are useful for presenting data because they allow the reader to understand the data visually. However, we lose some detail in the data when it is displayed graphically, especially around the distribution of data that are measured at the interval and ratio level (continuous variables).

When the data are measured at the interval or ratio level, it is important to present the distribution of data in terms of **central tendency** (i.e., the average case) and **variability** (i.e., the range and spread of the data from the center). For example, **Figure 6-1** shows a histogram of incomes of recent graduates in family nurse practitioner (FNP) programs. Questions we might ask about graduates are, "What would be the typical or average measurement value if one person was selected at random from this group?" and "How far from the average are data values spread?" These are difficult questions to answer with visual displays such as graphs, charts, and tables. We need numerical measures of central tendency and variability so that we can understand the distribution of the data on an objective basis.

These numeric measurements of central tendency and variability are examples of **descriptive statistics** and they help us to explain the data more accurately and in greater detail than graphical displays. However, it is always good to begin with graphical displays of the data to visually inspect the distribution; you should then confirm what was seen in the graphical displays with numeric descriptive statistics.

Data can be distributed in many different ways depending upon where the average is located and how the data values differ. The center of the distribution can be located in the middle, but it may be shifted to the left or right. The data can present with a high peak, where most of the data values are close to each other, but they may be far different from each other. Many statistical procedures we will discuss in later

Figure 6-1

Histogram of incomes of recent graduates in family nurse practitioner (FNP) programs.

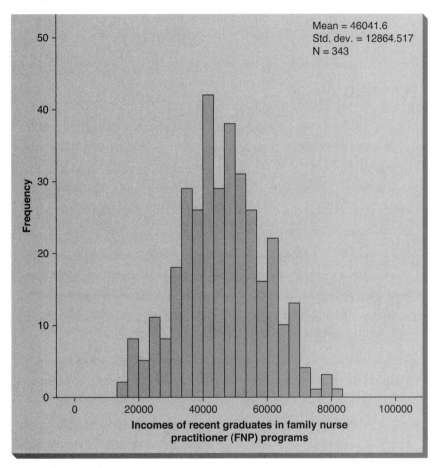

chapters assume that the data follow **normal distribution**, in which the percentages of data values are equal from the center of the distribution. Therefore, it is important to understand the characteristics of the normal distribution.

We will present how to compute measures of central tendency and variability and how to interpret them correctly to describe the data. We will also explain how descriptive statistics are used to understand normal distributions. Three common measures of central tendency—mode, mean, and median—will be explained first. Then, the four common measures of variability, range, interquartile range, variance, and standard deviation, are discussed, followed by the characteristics of normal distribution and confidence intervals. Let us begin with an example of the use of descriptive statistics from the real world.

Case Study

Dr. Huey-Ming Tzeng (2011) reported results from a study designed to explore the perceptions of patients and their visitors on the importance of and response time to call lights on general medical/surgical units in a Veterans Administration hospital. Dr. Tzeng noted that there is an established relationship between the use of call lights and the incidence of falls in acute care settings. The more patients use their call lights, the less likely falls are to occur. Dr. Tzeng was interested in finding out the reasons for and nature of patient- and family-initiated call lights, call light use, and response time to call lights. Such a study could provide a better understanding of call light use and support interventions to encourage call light use and improve response times.

Dr. Tzeng used descriptive statistics, measures of central tendency, and measures of variation to describe the results from the study. For example, Dr. Tzeng found that, on average, patients used their call light 3.66 times per day with a standard deviation of 2.96. We would understand that means a typical patient on a medical/surgical unit in this hospital used the call light about 3.66 times, and most of these patients (68%) used the call light between 0.70 times, and 6.62 times. Descriptive statistics, such as the arithmetic mean and the standard deviation, help us to understand both the typical case and the range of cases. Findings like this can be used by the researcher, advanced practice nurse, and nurse executive for a variety of purposes: evidence of the need for further research, support for improving practice, or assigning resources to manage a problem or support a solution.

MEASURES OF CENTRAL TENDENCY

The following are some of the example statements we can find in a newspaper and/or published journal articles.

The average annual premiums for employer-sponsored health insurance in 2011 are $5,429 for single coverage and $15,703 for family coverage (Kaiser Family Foundation, Health Research & Educational Trust, 2011).

The average job satisfaction rating for the study sample was 5.2 on a 7-point scale (Kovner et al., 2007).

The average blood pressure for all patients at the beginning of the study was 159/94 mmHg (Kershner, 2011).

All of these statements have used a single number to describe the data, and it helps us in understanding the data in terms of "average." There are multiple ways of computing and presenting averages, but we will describe the three most commonly used measures of **central tendency**: mode, median, and mean.

The Mode

The **mode** is simply the most frequently occurring number in a given data set. For example, let us take a look at the following data set of seven systolic blood pressure (SBP) measurements:

$$120 \quad 114 \quad 116 \quad 117 \quad 114 \quad 121 \quad 124$$

Notice that 114 appears twice, where the other measurements appear only one time. Therefore, the SBP measurement of 114 will be the mode in this data set since it is the most frequently occurring value. This distribution is called **unimodal distribution** since there is only one mode. Note, however, that it is possible to have more than one mode in a given data set. To explain, let us take a look at the following data set:

$$117 \quad 120 \quad 114 \quad 116 \quad 117 \quad 114 \quad 121 \quad 124$$

This data set has two modes, 114 and 117, since they each appear twice where the others appear only once. When a data set has two modes, it is known as **bimodal distribution**; a **multimodal distribution** is a distribution with more than two modes in a data set.

As you probably noticed by now, the mode is useful primarily for variables measured at the nominal level since it is merely the most frequently occurring number in the data set. For example, if we have assigned the following numbers to the sex of participants, 1 for men and 2 for women, and out of a sample of 100 there are 75 women, the mode is 2. The mode will not be useful with continuous levels of measurement, or as the data set gets larger.

The Mean

The arithmetic **mean** (often called the average) is the sum of all data values in a data set divided by the number of data values and is shown in the following equation:

$$Mean = \frac{Sum\ of\ all\ data\ values}{Number\ of\ data\ values}$$

The mean involves the minor mathematical operations of addition and division, and so is not an appropriate measure of central tendency for nominal levels of measurement. For example, it is impossible to find the mean for the variable *political affiliations*, with categories of Republican, Independent, and Democratic. The interpretation of the mean will only make sense when a variable's measurements can be quantifiable, such as in interval and ratio levels of measurement.

Let us consider the following data set of sodium content levels measured in milligrams per liter:

$$20 \quad 18 \quad 16 \quad 22 \quad 27 \quad 11$$

For this data set, the mean will be

$$Mean = \frac{(20 + 18 + 16 + 22 + 27 + 11)}{6} = 19$$

We have computed a mean of 19 for a group of 6 sodium content levels. How should we interpret this finding? Remember, the mean is the average score in the data set. Therefore, the mean of 19 tells us that there is, on average, 19 mg of sodium per liter in the data set.

The Median

The **median** is the exact middle value in a distribution, which divides the data set into two exact halves. Let us consider the following data set, which consists of five income levels for registered nurses:

35,000   39,500   42,000   47,500   52,000

In this data set, the value of 42,000 is the median, since it divides the data set into exactly two halves with an equal number of values below and above it.

Notice the data set is ordered from the smallest to the largest data value. However, correctly finding the middle value may be difficult and misleading if the data values are not ordered consecutively. Consider the following data set:

47,500   39,500   32,000   52,500   42,000

It will not make sense to choose 32,000 and report it as the median, since it is the smallest data value in this data set. Therefore, ordering the data from the smallest to the largest (or vice versa) is the first and the most important step in finding the median of any given data set. After ordering, it is easy to see that the median for this data set should be 42,000.

Notice also that the previous two data files had odd numbers of data values. Finding the median in a data set with an odd number of values is easy since you will end up with an equal number of data values above and below the median. However, it is less straightforward to find the median when there are an even number of data values in the data set. Let us take a look at the following data set:

24   29   32   35   39   40

The data values represent age in years of six individuals, and there is no such number that divides this data set into two exact halves. Theoretically, such a number should be between 32 and 35, leaving three data values above and below it. However, such a number does not actually exist in the data set. In this case, you will sum the two middle numbers, 32 and 35, and divide the sum by 2. You are basically computing the average of those two middle values as the median, which is:

$$\frac{32 + 35}{2} = 33.5$$

This value of 33.5 as the median makes sense since we have an equal number of data values above and below it.

Choosing a Measure of Central Tendency

We have discussed three ~~types of central tendency—the mode, the mean, and the median~~—and examined how they differ in terms of finding the center of a data distribution. The next legitimate question to ask may be "When do we use which measure?"

The ~~mode is simply the most frequently occurring data value~~(s) ~~in the data set. Therefore, it is mainly useful for the nominal level of measurement~~. Both ~~median and mean are useful when the variable being measured can be quantified~~. However, one important thing to note here is that the mean is extremely sensitive to unusual cases. To explain this further, let us consider the following data sets:

Data set #1:   108   112   116   120   124

Data set #2:   108   112   116   120   205

In both data sets, the median is 116, as it is the number that divides the data set into two exact halves. However, you will notice that the mean is not identical in both data sets. For the first data set, the mean is equal to

$$\frac{108 + 112 + 116 + 120 + 124}{5} = 116$$

where the mean of the second data set is equal to

$$\frac{108 + 112 + 116 + 120 + 205}{5} = 132.2$$

Notice how the mean of the second data set has been influenced by the presence of an unusual case in the data set. If we were to say the mean is equal to 132.5 for the second data set and it represents a typical case, this will not make much sense because the majority of data values are less than 120. Therefore, the mean should not be used when unusual, or outlying, data values are present in the data set, as the mean tends to be extremely sensitive to the unusual values. Rather, the median should be reported in this case. This is why the average housing price is always reported with the median, since even one million-dollar house can distort the average housing price when most of the houses are in the $200,000–$350,000 range.

MEASURES OF VARIABILITY

Measures of central tendency allow us to know the typical value in the data set. However, we know that when we measure a variable, there will be differences between and among the values in the data set. For example, if we were measuring systolic blood pressure among a group of research participants, we would expect that there would be a range of values between individuals. Furthermore, we would expect similar variation on systolic blood pressure measurements in any given individual participant. In other words, some level of **variation** among data values in any data set is expected. Given this expected variation, we might ask, "How accurate is the measure of central tendency?" The computed measure of central tendency will be most accurate when the data values vary only a little, but accuracy of the mean declines as the variation in data values increases. Measures of variability provide information about the spread of scores and indicate how well a measure of central tendency represents the "middle/average" value in the data set. There are multiple ways of computing and presenting variability, but we describe the four that are most commonly used: range, interquartile range, variance, and standard deviation.

Range   *Very sensitive*

Range is the difference between the largest and the smallest values in the data set. For example, suppose a researcher measured patients' level of pain after vascular surgery on a scale of 1 to 10. These data are shown below.

$$9 \quad 3 \quad 2 \quad 6 \quad 7 \quad 8 \quad 7 \quad 5$$

The first step is to sort the data from the smallest to the largest values, as it will make our job of finding these two values easy. After sorting, the range of this data set is $9 - 2 = 7$.

Range is simple to calculate. However, we should be cautious about using range as a measure of variability. As seen in the previous example, the range is calculated simply by subtracting the smallest value from the highest value. In addition, it allows us to understand what the collected data set looks like. However, the range is a very crude measure of variability as it only uses the highest and lowest values in computation. Therefore, it does not accurately capture information about how data values in the set differ if the data set contains an unusual value(s).

Consider the following data set.

3   4   2   3   3   4   2   9

This data set is still a collection of pain level measurements of patients who underwent vascular surgery, but notice that the value of 9 seems unusual in this data set. Here, the range is $9 - 2 = 7$ after sorting. Does this make sense? Most of the values are between 2 and 4, and claiming the variability is 7 does not really make sense in the context of this data set. It is clear that the range is extremely sensitive to the unusual data values. To get around this problem, sometimes researchers will simply report the range as the lowest and highest values, "reports of pain intensity ranged from three to nine," rather than computing a range.

Interquartile Range

Interquartile range is the difference between the 75th percentile and 25th percentile. As we saw in Chapter 5, the percentile is a measure of location and tells us how many data values fall below a certain percentage of observations. Therefore, the 25th percentile is the data value that the bottom 25% falls below and the 75th percentile is the data value that the bottom 75% falls below. In results, the interquartile range is less sensitive to an unusual case(s) in the data set as it does not use the smallest and the largest value. For example, suppose the number of patient falls per week at a local nursing home have been measured.

1   1   2   2   2   3   3   3   4   4   5

Note that the data set has already been sorted from the smallest to the largest. It is easier to find the median first and then to find 25th and 75th percentiles, since it less straightforward to directly identify the percentiles.

The median of this data set is 3, since 3 is the exact middle that divides this data set into two exact halves. From the median, the 25th percentile is equal to 2 and the 75th percentile is equal to 4, as they divide the lower and upper halves of the data set into two exact halves, respectively. The interquartile range is then the difference between the 25th percentile and the 75th percentile, which is $4 - 2 = 2$.

Let us now consider the next data set.

$$1 \quad 1 \quad 2 \quad 2 \quad 2 \quad 3 \quad 3 \quad 3 \quad 4 \quad 4 \quad 24$$

As you can see, it is the same data set as before, except for the highest value, 24, which seems to be an unusual value. Notice that the interquartile range is still $4 - 2 = 2$ and is not affected by the unusual data value. Therefore, interquartile range is not as sensitive to unusual or outlying values as the standard range.

Variance and Standard Deviation

While range provides a rough estimate of the variability of a data set, it does not use all of the data values in computation and is very sensitive to an unusual value in the data set. Interquartile range is an improvement, but still does not account for every data value in the set. On the other hand, the next two measures of variability, variance and standard deviation, use all of the data values in the set in computation and may capture information about variability more precisely than the range or the interquartile range. As **standard deviation** is simply the square root of variance, we will explain variance first.

Variance is the average amount that data values differ from the mean and is computed with the following formula:

$$Population \; variance = \frac{\Sigma(X - \mu)^2}{N}$$

$$Sample \; variance = \frac{\Sigma(X - \overline{X})^2}{n - 1}$$

In this equation we compute the difference between each raw value and the mean $(X - \overline{X})$, square it, sum (Σ) those values and then divide by the total number of values in the data set (N). Note that the denominator will be changed to $n - 1$ when working with samples.

Degrees of Freedom

Calculations of variance and many other statistics require an estimate of the range of variability, known as **degrees of freedom**. From a sample, degrees of freedom are always equal to $n - 1$. Here is an analogy that might help: Envision a beverage holder from any fast food restaurant—most of these hold four drinks. In this case, the degrees of freedom would be equal to $4 - 1$, or 3. As each section of the holder is occupied by a drink, there is a chance of varying in what section of the holder any given drink is placed, top left or top right for example, until three of the sections are filled; at this point, there is only one section left where a drink may be placed and no variation is possible.

Each statistical test or calculation has a variation of degrees of freedom. Watch for these throughout the text.

Consider the following data set of toddler weights in an outpatient clinic to explain how to compute the variance, assuming that the data values were taken from a population:

$$17 \quad 12 \quad 14 \quad 16 \quad 19$$

The computation steps are shown in **Table 6-1**.

Computed variance for this data set is 5.84. What does this mean? In fact, we cannot use this as a measure of variability. Let us assume that the values represent weight losses measured in pounds taken from five subjects. Because the deviation of each observation from the mean has been squared, the unit for the variance is now in $(pound)^2$. What does $(pound)^2$ mean? If we were to say that data values differ from the mean on average about 5.84 $(pound)^2$, would this claim make sense? Probably not, since there is no such unit as a $(pound)^2$.

Why do we then take the square of the deviation if the $(unit)^2$ will not make sense to interpret at the end? The answer is simple: If you do not square the deviation and sum each deviation, it will always add up to zero no matter what data set you work with. We suggest you to try this with small data sets you can find in this text or other sources.

Table

6-1 How to Compute the Variance

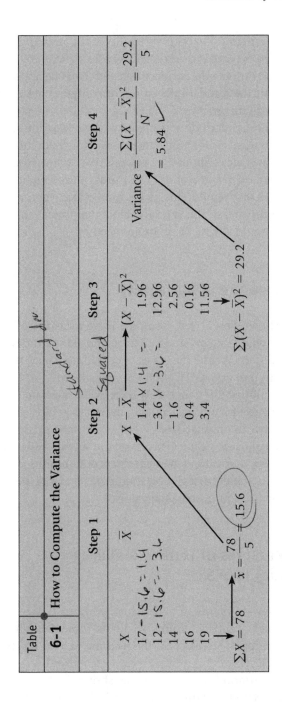

standard dev

Step 1	Step 2	Step 3	Step 4
$\overline{X}$	$X - \overline{X}$ →	$(X - \overline{X})^2$	$\text{Variance} = \dfrac{\Sigma(X - \overline{X})^2}{N} = \dfrac{29.2}{5}$

X

17 − 15.6 = 1.4

12 − 15.6 = −3.6

14

16

19

$\Sigma X = 78$ → $\overline{X} = \dfrac{78}{5} = 15.6$

Step 2: 1.4 × 1.4 =

−3.6 × −3.6 =

−1.6

0.4

3.4

Step 3 (Squared):

1.96

12.96

2.56

0.16

11.56

$\Sigma(X - \overline{X})^2 = 29.2$

Step 4: $= 5.84$ ✓

How can we then talk about variability if the measure of variability comes out to be equal to zero? This is why we take the square of the deviation to compute the variance first and then take the square root of it to compute the standard deviation, bringing us back to the original unit of measurement.

We get the standard deviation of 2.42 by taking the square root of 5.84; we can then say that the data values differ from the mean (15.60 lbs.) on an average of about 2.42 pounds. We can interpret this finding to mean that, on average, about two thirds of the weights fall between 13.18 and 18.02 pounds. This makes more sense when you look at the data set, compared to the variance. Note that the mean and standard deviation should always be reported together!

Choosing a Measure of Variability

We have shown you how to compute three measures of variability—range, interquatile range, and variation and standard deviation—and how they differ. Like the measures of central tendency, the next legitimate question to ask is, "When do we use which?"

You should use the range only as a crude measure, since it is extremely sensitive to unusual values in the data set. Interquartile range is not as sensitive to unusual data values, where standard deviation is very sensitive to unusual values. Therefore, the interquartile range should be used with the median when the data contain unusual data values. However, the standard deviation should be used with the mean when the data are free of unusual data values.

Obtaining Measures of Central Tendency and Variability in SPSS

There are several places in SPSS where you can request measures of central tendency and variability. To obtain these measures, go to Analyze > Descriptive Statistics. In the next menu, choose "Frequencies" (**Figure 6-2**).

Move a variable(s) of interest, as shown in **Figure 6-3**. Of the three buttons on the right side of the window, select "Statistics" (see

Figure 6-2

Selecting the Frequency window in SPSS.

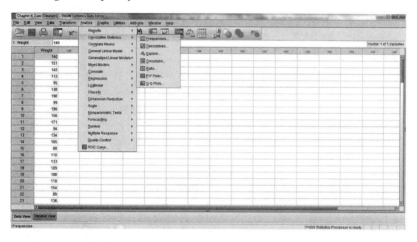

Figure 6-4). You can select measures of both central tendency and variability to obtain the measures to suit your needs.

The same measures can be obtained by choosing "Descriptives" or "Explore" under the Analyze > Descriptive Statistics pull-down menu. Note also that these measures of central tendency and variability can be obtained within windows for several other statistical procedures.

Figure 6-3

The Frequency window in SPSS.

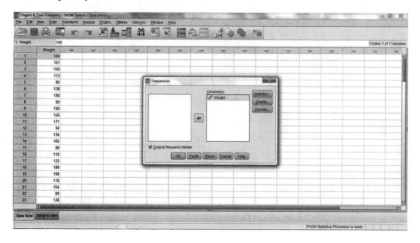

button in the Frequency window.

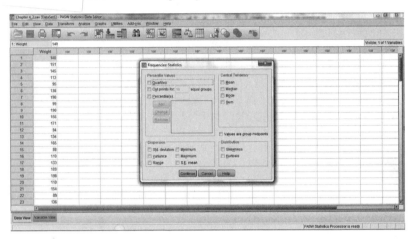

NORMAL DISTRIBUTION

Descriptive statistics helps us understand whether the distribution of a continuously measured variable is normal. **Figure 6-5** is an example normal distribution of a variable, age. Some notable characteristics of normal distribution are summarized below.

Characteristics of Normal Distribution

- It is bell-shaped and symmetric.
- The area under a normal curve is equal to 1.00 or 100%.
- 68% of observations fall within one standard deviation from the mean in both directions.
- 95% of observations fall within two standard deviations from the mean in both directions.
- 99.7% of observations fall within three standard deviations from the mean in both directions.
- Many normal distributions exist with different means and standard deviations.

Figure 6-5

Histogram with overlying normal curve.

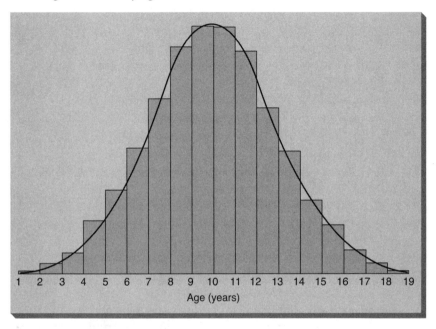

When a normal distribution is said to be symmetrical, it means that the area on both sides of the distribution from the mean is equal; in other words, 50% of the data values in the set are smaller than the mean and the other 50% are larger than the mean. In a normal distribution, the mean is located at the highest peak of the distribution and the spread of a normal distribution can be presented in terms of the standard deviation.

No data will ever be exactly/perfectly normally distributed in reality. If that is so, how do we know whether or not a collected data set is normally distributed? We can begin with a visual display of the data in a histogram to see if the data set is normally distributed. However, a visual check, alone, may not be sufficient to know whether the data are normally distributed. There are statistical measures, **skewness and kurtosis**, which, along with a histogram, allow us to determine whether the set is normally distributed. Skewness is a measure of whether the set is symmetrical or off-center, which means probabilities on both sides of the distribution are not the same. Kurtosis is a measure of how

Figure 6-6

Area under a normal distribution.

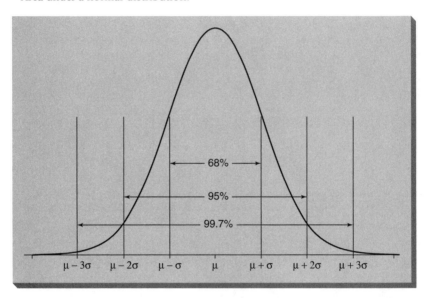

peaked a distribution is. A distribution is said to be normal when both measures of skewness and kurtosis fall between −1 and +1 range and nonnormal if both measures fall either below −1 or above +1. Note that these measures can be selected in the same window as measures of central tendency and variability, which we just discussed.

Figure 6-6 shows what percentage of the set falls within how many standard deviations away from the mean. If a variable follows a normal distribution, these rules can be applied to understand the distribution of the variable in terms of the mean and the standard deviation. In addition, different normal distributions can be found when the mean and the standard deviation are defined as shown in **Figure 6-7** and **Figure 6-8**.

Why do we care about this normal distribution so much? The most important reason is that many human characteristics fall into an approximately normal distribution and that the measurement scores are assumed to be normally distributed when running most statistical analyses. Therefore, the statistical results you get at the end may not be trustworthy if the variable is not normally distributed. We will discuss this more in Chapter 8.

Figure 6-7

Normal distributions with different means.

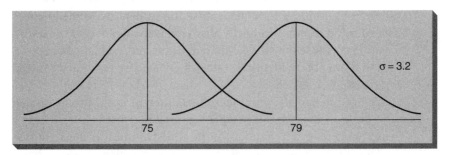

Let us consider an example where a student looks at her final exam scores in her statistics and research courses. The student scored 79 out of 100 on the final exam in the statistics course and 42 out of 60 on the final exam in the research course. Can the student conclude that her performance was better in statistics because of the higher score in the statistics course than the research course? Before making such a conclusion, the student will need to examine the distribution of scores on the two final exams. Let us assume that the final exam in statistics

Figure 6-8

Normal distributions with different standard deviations.

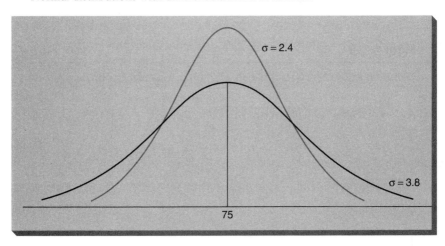

had a mean of 75 with a standard deviation of 3, and the final exam in research had a mean of 40 with a standard deviation of 2.5. It seems that the student did better than the average in both classes, but it is still difficult to judge in which course the student performed better. This question cannot be directly answered using different normal distributions because they have different means and standard deviations (i.e., they are not on identical scale, which is necessary to make direct comparisons).

We need to somehow put these two different distributions on the same scale so that we can make a legitimate comparison of the student's performance; a **standard normal distribution** is the solution. By definition, a normal distribution is one in which all scores have been put on the same scale (standardized). These standardized scores (also known as z-scores) represent how far below or above the mean a given score falls and allows us to determine percentile/probabilities associated with a given score.

Figure 6-9 shows a graphical transition from a general normal distribution to a standard normal distribution. Characteristics of the standard normal distribution are summarized in the box on the next page.

To compute a z-score, you will need two pieces of information about a distribution: the mean and the standard deviation. **Z-scores (standardized scores)** are computed using the following equation and calculated such that positive values indicate how far above the mean a score falls and negative values indicate how far below the mean a score falls. Whether positive or negative, larger z-scores mean that scores are

Figure 6-9

Transition from a general normal distribution to a standard normal distribution.

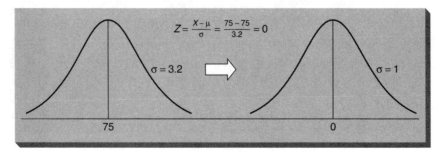

Characteristics of the Standard Normal Distribution

- The standard normal distribution has a mean of 0 and standard deviation of 1.
- The area under the standard normal curve is equal to 1 or 100%.
- Z-scores have associated probabilities, which are fixed and known.

far away from the mean, and smaller z-scores mean that scores are close to the mean.

$$Z = \frac{X - \mu}{\sigma}$$

Where the population mean (μ) is subtracted from the raw score and divided by the population standard deviation (σ). When do you think z-scores will be computed with positive or negative sign? Z-scores will be positive when a student performs better than the mean on a test—the numerator of the equation above will be positive and will be above the mean. On the other hand, z-scores will be negative when a student performs below the mean. Let us consider an example test, again a statistics final exam, with a mean of 78 and standard deviation of 3. Suppose Brian has a final exam score of 84. His z-score will be

$$Z = \frac{X - \mu}{\sigma} = \frac{84 - 78}{3} = 2$$

What does Brian's z-score of 2 mean in terms of his performance relative to the average person who took this statistics final exam? First, we can see that Brian did perform better than the average person on this final exam. Second, his z-score of 2 tells us that his score is two standard deviations above the average score of 78 since a standard normal distribution has a standard deviation of 1. However, this second point about Brian's score does not really make perfect sense to us yet. From **Figure 6-10**, we can see that Brian seems to have performed better than a number of students in his class. However, we still do not know exactly how much better he did. To find out the exact percentile

Figure 6-10

Brian's z-score.

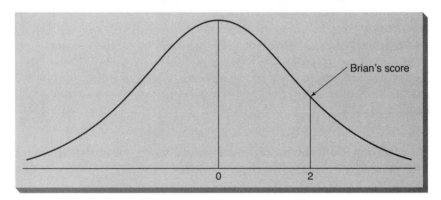

rank of another student, Sam, we need to use a z table, shown in **Figure 6-11**. Steps in using the z table to find a corresponding percentile rank are summarized in the box at the bottom of this page.

Let us consider another example that will help us understand how to find the corresponding probability for a given score. The sodium intakes for a group of obese patients at a local hospital are known to have a mean of 4,500 mg/day and a standard deviation of $+/-150$ mg/day. Assuming that the sodium intake is normally distributed, let us find the probability that a randomly selected obese patient will have a sodium intake level below 4,275 mg/day. First, we need

---

Using the z Table to Find a Corresponding Percentile Rank of a Score

1. Convert Brian's final exam score to a corresponding z-score.
2. Locate the row in the z table for a z-score of $+2.00$. Note that the z-scores in the first column are shown in only the first decimal. Locate also the column for .00 so that you get 2.00 when you add 2.0 and .00.
3. Brian's z-score of $+2.00$ gives probabilities of .9772 to the left.
4. Therefore, Brian's final exam score of $+2.00$ corresponds to the 98th percentile. Brian did better than 98% of the students in the class.

Figure 6-11

z table. *Source:* Gerstman, B. (2008). *Basic biostatistics: Statistics for public health practice.* Sudbury, MA: Jones and Barlett.

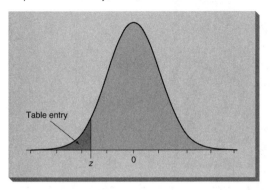

z	hundredths									
tenths	.00	.01	.02	.03	.04	.05	.06	.07	.08	.09
−3.4	.0003	.0003	.0003	.0003	.0003	.0003	.0003	.0003	.0003	.0002
−3.3	.0005	.0005	.0005	.0004	.0004	.0004	.0004	.0004	.0004	.0003
−3.2	.0007	.0007	.0006	.0006	.0006	.0006	.0006	.0005	.0005	.0005
−3.1	.0010	.0009	.0009	.0009	.0008	.0008	.0008	.0008	.0007	.0007
−3.0	.0013	.0013	.0013	.0012	.0012	.0011	.0011	.0011	.0010	.0010
−2.9	.0019	.0018	.0018	.0017	.0016	.0016	.0015	.0015	.0014	.0014
−2.8	.0026	.0025	.0024	.0023	.0023	.0022	.0021	.0021	.0020	.0019
−2.7	.0035	.0034	.0033	.0032	.0031	.0030	.0029	.0028	.0027	.0026
−2.6	.0047	.0045	.0044	.0043	.0041	.0040	.0039	.0038	.0037	.0036
−2.5	.0062	.0060	.0059	.0057	.0055	.0054	.0052	.0051	.0049	.0048
−2.4	.0082	.0080	.0078	.0075	.0073	.0071	.0069	.0068	.0066	.0064
−2.3	.0107	.0104	.0102	.0099	.0096	.0094	.0091	.0089	.0087	.0084
−2.2	.0139	.0136	.0132	.0129	.0125	.0122	.0119	.0116	.0113	.0110
−2.1	.0179	.0174	.0170	.0166	.0162	.0158	.0154	.0150	.0146	.0143
−2.0	.0228	.0222	.0217	.0212	.0207	.0202	.0197	.0192	.0188	.0183
−1.9	.0287	.0281	.0274	.0268	.0262	.0256	.0250	.0244	.0239	.0233
−1.8	.0359	.0351	.0344	.0336	.0329	.0322	.0314	.0307	.0301	.0294
−1.7	.0446	.0436	.0427	.0418	.0409	.0401	.0392	.0384	.0375	.0367
−1.6	.0548	.0537	.0526	.0516	.0505	.0495	.0485	.0475	.0465	.0455
−1.5	.0668	.0655	.0643	.0630	.0618	.0606	.0594	.0582	.0571	.0559
−1.4	.0808	.0793	.0778	.0764	.0749	.0735	.0721	.0708	.0694	.0681
−1.3	.0968	.0951	.0934	.0918	.0901	.0885	.0869	.0853	.0838	.0823
−1.2	.1151	.1131	.1112	.1093	.1075	.1056	.1038	.1020	.1003	.0985
−1.1	.1357	.1335	.1314	.1292	.1271	.1251	.1230	.1210	.1190	.1170
−1.0	.1587	.1562	.1539	.1515	.1492	.1469	.1446	.1423	.1401	.1379
−0.9	.1841	.1814	.1788	.1762	.1736	.1711	.1685	.1660	.1635	.1611
−0.8	.2119	.2090	.2061	.2033	.2005	.1977	.1949	.1922	.1894	.1867
−0.7	.2420	.2389	.2358	.2327	.2296	.2266	.2236	.2206	.2177	.2148
−0.6	.2743	.2709	.2676	.2643	.2611	.2578	.2546	.2514	.2483	.2451
−0.5	.3085	.3050	.3015	.2981	.2946	.2912	.2877	.2843	.2810	.2776
−0.4	.3446	.3409	.3372	.3336	.3300	.3264	.3228	.3192	.3156	.3121
−0.3	.3821	.3783	.3745	.3707	.3669	.3632	.3594	.3557	.3520	.3483
−0.2	.4207	.4168	.4129	.4090	.4052	.4013	.3974	.3936	.3897	.3859
−0.1	.4602	.4562	.4522	.4483	.4443	.4404	.4364	.4325	.4286	.4247
−0.0	.5000	.4960	.4920	.4880	.4840	.4801	.4761	.4721	.4681	.4641

Cumulative probabilities computed with Microsoft Excel 9.0 NORMSDIST function.

(continues)

Figure 6-11

Continued

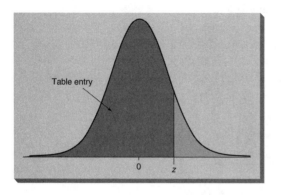

z	hundredths									
tenths	.00	.01	.02	.03	.04	.05	.06	.07	.08	.09
0.0	.5000	.5040	.5080	.5120	.5160	.5199	.5239	.5279	.5319	.5359
0.1	.5398	.5438	.5478	.5517	.5557	.5596	.5636	.5675	.5714	.5753
0.2	.5793	.5832	.5871	.5910	.5948	.5987	.6026	.6064	.6103	.6141
0.3	.6179	.6217	.6255	.6293	.6331	.6368	.6406	.6443	.6480	.6517
0.4	.6554	.6591	.6628	.6664	.6700	.6736	.6772	.6808	.6844	.6879
0.5	.6915	.6950	.6985	.7019	.7054	.7088	.7123	.7157	.7190	.7224
0.6	.7257	.7291	.7324	.7357	.7389	.7422	.7454	.7486	.7517	.7549
0.7	.7580	.7611	.7642	.7673	.7704	.7734	.7764	.7794	.7823	.7852
0.8	.7881	.7910	.7939	.7967	.7995	.8023	.8051	.8078	.8106	.8133
0.9	.8159	.8186	.8212	.8238	.8264	.8289	.8315	.8340	.8365	.8389
1.0	.8413	.8438	.8461	.8485	.8508	.8531	.8554	.8577	.8599	.8621
1.1	.8643	.8665	.8686	.8708	.8729	.8749	.8770	.8790	.8810	.8830
1.2	.8849	.8869	.8888	.8907	.8925	.8944	.8962	.8980	.8997	.9015
1.3	.9032	.9049	.9066	.9082	.9099	.9115	.9131	.9147	.9162	.9177
1.4	.9192	.9207	.9222	.9236	.9251	.9265	.9279	.9292	.9306	.9319
1.5	.9332	.9345	.9357	.9370	.9382	.9394	.9406	.9418	.9429	.9441
1.6	.9452	.9463	.9474	.9484	.9495	.9505	.9515	.9525	.9535	.9545
1.7	.9554	.9564	.9573	.9582	.9591	.9599	.9608	.9616	.9625	.9633
1.8	.9641	.9649	.9656	.9664	.9671	.9678	.9686	.9693	.9699	.9706
1.9	.9713	.9719	.9726	.9732	.9738	.9744	.9750	.9756	.9761	.9767
2.0	.9772	.9778	.9783	.9788	.9793	.9798	.9803	.9808	.9812	.9817
2.1	.9821	.9826	.9830	.9834	.9838	.9842	.9846	.9850	.9854	.9857
2.2	.9861	.9864	.9868	.9871	.9875	.9878	.9881	.9884	.9887	.9890
2.3	.9893	.9896	.9898	.9901	.9904	.9906	.9909	.9911	.9913	.9916
2.4	.9918	.9920	.9922	.9925	.9927	.9929	.9931	.9932	.9934	.9936
2.5	.9938	.9940	.9941	.9943	.9945	.9946	.9948	.9949	.9951	.9952
2.6	.9953	.9955	.9956	.9957	.9959	.9960	.9961	.9962	.9963	.9964
2.7	.9965	.9966	.9967	.9968	.9969	.9970	.9971	.9972	.9973	.9974
2.8	.9974	.9975	.9976	.9977	.9977	.9978	.9979	.9979	.9980	.9981
2.9	.9981	.9982	.9982	.9983	.9984	.9984	.9985	.9985	.9986	.9986
3.0	.9987	.9987	.9987	.9988	.9988	.9989	.9989	.9989	.9990	.9990
3.1	.9990	.9991	.9991	.9991	.9992	.9992	.9992	.9992	.9993	.9993
3.2	.9993	.9993	.9994	.9994	.9994	.9994	.9994	.9995	.9995	.9995
3.3	.9995	.9995	.9995	.9996	.9996	.9996	.9996	.9996	.9996	.9997
3.4	.9997	.9997	.9997	.9997	.9997	.9997	.9997	.9997	.9997	.9998

to convert this value into the *z*-score. The corresponding *z*-score for 4,275 mg/day will be

$$Z = \frac{X - \mu}{\sigma} = \frac{4275 - 4500}{150} = -1.5$$

Locating the row in the *z* table for a *z*-score of −1.5 and the column for .00, you should get a probability of .0668. Therefore, the probability that a randomly selected obese patient will take in below 4,275 mg/day will be 6.68%. How about the probability that a randomly selected obese patient will have between 4,350 mg/day and 4,725 mg/day? Notice here that we have two scores to transform. The corresponding *z*-score of the lower level, 4,350 mg/day, will be

$$Z = \frac{X - \mu}{\sigma} = \frac{4350 - 4500}{150} = -1$$

and the upper level, 4,725 mg/day, will be

$$Z = \frac{X - \mu}{\sigma} = \frac{4725 - 4500}{150} = +1.5$$

Therefore, we are looking at the area under the normal curve between −1 and +1.5 standard deviations, as shown in **Figure 6-12**. The probability to the left of +1.5 is .9332 and the probability to the left of −1 is .1587. To get the probability between −1 and +1.5, we will subtract

Figure 6-12

The normal curve between −1 and +1.5 standard deviations.

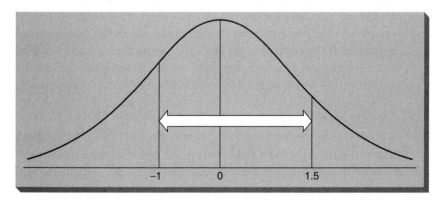

.1587 from .9332 and should get .7745. Therefore, the probability that a randomly selected obese patient will have a sodium intake between 4,350 mg/day and 4,725 mg/day will be 77.45%. Finding the corresponding probabilities for a given score can be tricky, so we recommend you work on as many as examples as you can, including what we provide you at the end of this chapter.

As a closing note about the standard normal distribution, recall that the following are true when a variable is normally distributed:

- 68% of observations fall within one standard deviation from the mean in both directions
- 95% of observations fall within two standard deviations from the mean in both directions
- 99.7% of observations fall within three standard deviations from the mean in both directions.

This means that 68% of the z-scores will fall between -1 and $+1$, 95% of the z-scores will fall between -2 and $+2$, and 99.7% of the z-scores will fall between -3 and $+3$, since the standard normal distribution has a mean of 0 and a standard deviation of 1. This is important because any z-score that is greater than $+3$ or less than -3 can be treated as unusual.

CONFIDENCE INTERVAL

Up to this point, all of the estimates we calculated were with a single number. Measures of both central tendency and variability were a single number and allowed us to say that those measures are the average measurements and the spread of values on average of a given variable, respectively. These are called **point estimates**. However, we may not be lucky enough to hit exactly what the actual average will be in the population, since we are likely to use a sample taken from the population. In other words, we will never be sure that our estimates will accurately reflect values in the population as a whole, as shown in **Figure 6-13**.

To deal with this problem, we can create boundaries that we think the population mean will fall between, instead of computing a single estimate from a sample; these boundaries are called **confidence intervals**. It is another way of answering an important question, "How

Figure 6-13

Different sample means from a population.

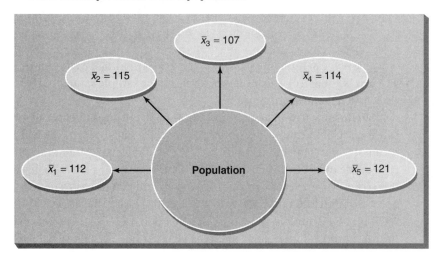

well does the sample statistic represent the unknown population parameter?"

Confidence intervals use confidence levels in the computation. Confidence level is determined by the researcher and reflects how accurate you want to be in computing a confidence interval as a percentage. There are three confidence levels that you can choose from: 90%, 95%, and 99% (although the 95% confidence level seems to be the most popular choice). What does confidence interval mean? Let us say that you chose a 95% confidence level to compute a confidence interval; this means that if you were to compute 100 confidence intervals, 95 of those confidence intervals will contain the population parameter and 5 of those will not. Another way of thinking about it is to say that should we calculate 100 confidence intervals, 5 of those would likely not be accurate. There are different equations for different parameters in the computation of confidence intervals, but we will introduce only one here for a population mean and focus on how to interpret the computed confidence interval.

Let us assume that you are a health researcher and would like to investigate the average number of hours nursing students at a local university spent per week studying for statistics. The number of hours is measured on the ratio level of measurement, and we are looking at the mean hours. Since we need to compute a confidence interval for the mean, we will use the following equation:

$$\bar{x} - z_{\alpha/2}\frac{s}{\sqrt{n}} < \mu < \bar{x} + z_{\alpha/2}\frac{s}{\sqrt{n}}$$

where $\bar{x}$ is the sample mean, $z_{\alpha/2}$ is the corresponding z-value for $\alpha/2$ where α is equal to $1 -$ confidence level, s is the sample standard deviation, and n is the sample size.

Let us assume that we obtained a sample of 30 nursing students and the distribution of the number of hours they study for statistics per week had a mean of 8 and standard deviation of 2. We would like to compute a 90% confidence interval where $z_{\alpha/2} = 1.645$. Our α is .10 since we are using a 90% confidence level and $\alpha/2$ is .05. We will find that the corresponding z-score for the closest probability to .95 $(1 - .05)$ inside the z table is 1.64, 1.65, or 1.645 (middle value between 1.64 and 1.65 as we cannot find the exact probability). Using 1.645, the 90% confidence interval will be:

$$8 - 1.645\frac{2}{\sqrt{30}} < \mu < 8 + 1.645\frac{2}{\sqrt{30}}$$

$$7.3993 < \mu < 8.6007$$

We can conclude from this finding that 90% of the time the mean will fall between 7.40 and 8.60 hours of studying for statistics.

Consider now that you would like to compute a 95% confidence interval for the same example above. Our $z_{\alpha/2}$ is 1.96 since our $\alpha/2$ is .025 for a 95% confidence level, and the 95% confidence interval will be:

$$8 - 1.96\frac{2}{\sqrt{30}} < \mu < 8 + 1.96\frac{2}{\sqrt{30}}$$

$$7.2843 < \mu < 8.7157$$

In this case we can conclude that 95% of the time the mean hours of studying for statistics fall between 7.28 and 8.72.

How about a 99% confidence interval for the same example? Our $z_{\alpha/2}$ is 2.58 since our $\alpha/2$ is .005 for a 99% confidence level and the 99% confidence interval will be:

$$8 - 2.58\frac{2}{\sqrt{30}} < \mu < 8 + 2.58\frac{2}{\sqrt{30}}$$

$$7.0579 < \mu < 8.9421$$

In this example we can conclude that 99% (
that students spend studying for statistics is

As you look at these three confidence inte
the confidence interval gets wider as your (
increases. This makes sense since the wider i
the more you are sure that the interval will i
parameter. The trade-off is that as confiden(...creases, the
likelihood of the confidence interval including a true population
parameter increases.

SUMMARY

Descriptive statistics, such as measures of central tendency and variability, help us to understand typical cases in a sample and the distribution
of a variable more clearly. Measures of central tendency include the
mode, the median, and the mean, and these provide us with an idea of
what may be the typical/average data value in the data set. The mode
should be used only for categorical data as it basically counts the frequencies. The median should be reported when an unusual data value
is present in the data set. Otherwise, the mean should be reported as it
possesses statistically preferable characteristics.

Measures of variability include the range, the interquartile range,
the variance, and the standard deviation, and they provide us an idea
of the accuracy of the measures of central tendency. The range should
be used as a crude measure of variability as it is extremely sensitive to
the presence of unusual data values. The interquartile range should be
reported when an unusual or outlying data value is present in the data
set. Otherwise, the standard deviation should be reported as it possesses statistically preferable characteristics.

A normal distribution is a very important probability distribution, which can represent many human characteristics, such as height,
weight, and blood pressure. Skewness and kurtosis can be used to
assess whether a variable is normally distributed; values should be
between -1 and $+1$ standard deviations to be normal. It is important
that variables of interest be normally distributed as most statistical
analyses assume a normal distribution.

When a variable is normally distributed, 68% of observations will
fall within one standard deviation from the mean, 95% of observations

will fall within two standard deviations from the mean, and 99.7% of observations will fall within three standard deviations from the mean. Any value that falls outside of the three standard deviation range can be treated as an unusual value for the data set.

Z-scores are a good example of how we can compute standardized scores to determine where any given score(s) fall in a normal distribution. We can use standardized scores to make comparisons between a single score, such as on a standardized test, with all scores.

Instead of estimating an unknown population parameter with a single number or point estimate, one can create an interval, called a confidence interval, as a different way of answering to the question, "How well does the sample statistic represent an unknown population parameter?" Confidence intervals are interpreted as the interval that will include the true parameter with a given confidence level, either 90%, 95%, or 99%. As the percentage of the confidence interval goes up (increased confidence that the mean falls within that range) the likelihood of confidence interval including a true population parameter increases.

Critical Thinking Questions www

1. What is the purpose of computing descriptive statistics? Why should we look at them along with graphical displays of a data set?
2. Which measure of central tendency and variability should be reported when an unusual data value is present in the data set? Explain.
3. The 95% confidence interval for sodium content level in 32 nursing home patients is (4,250 mg/day, 4,750 mg/day). What does this confidence interval tell us?

Self-Quiz www

1. True or false: Descriptive statistics are used to summarize about the sample and the measures in the data set.

2. True or false: The variance of length of stay at a local hospital is 25. The standard deviation is 5, and this is how each value differs on average from the mean.
3. True or false: There is no such chart that allows a researcher to identify possible outliers.
4. Which of the following is not measure of central tendency?
   a. Mode
   b. Interquartile range
   c. Mean
   d. Median
5. Find the area under the normal distribution curve.
   a. To the left of $z = -0.59$
   b. To the left of $z = 2.41$
   c. To the right of $z = -1.32$
   d. To the right of $z = 0.27$
   e. Between -0.87 and 0.87
   f. Between -2.99 and -1.34
6. The average time it takes for emergency nurses to respond to an emergency call is known to be 25 minutes. Assume the variable is approximately normally distributed and the standard deviation is 5 minutes. If we randomly select an emergency nurse, find the probability of the selected nurse responding to an emergency call in less than 20 minutes.
7. The average age of 25 local nursing home residents is known to be 72, and the standard deviation is 8. The director of the nursing home wants to compute a 95% confidence interval to understand the accuracy of an estimate for the average age of all residents. What is the 95% confidence interval?
   a. (65.23, 78.77)
   b. (68.86, 75.14)
   c. (65.00, 74.00)
   d. (62.86, 82.14)

REFERENCES

Kaiser Family Foundation, Health Research & Educational Trust. (2011). *Employer health benefit: 2011 annual survey.* Retrieved from http://ehbs.kff.org/pdf/8226.pdf

Kershner, K. (n.d.). *Drug effective against high blood pressure and prostate problems.* Retrieved from http://researchnews.osu.edu/archive/hytrin.htm

Kovner, C. T., Brewer, C. S., Fairchild, S., Poornima, S., Kim, H, & Djudic, M. (2007). Newly licensed RNs' characteristics, work ethics, and intentions to work. *American Journal of Nursing, 107*(9), 58–70.

Tzeng, H. (2011). Perspectives of patients and families about the nature of and reasons for call light use and staff call light response time. *Medsurg Nursing, 20*(5), 225–234.

Chapter

7 Hypothesis Testing

Learning Objectives

The principal goal of this chapter is to define the basic terminologies of hypothesis testing and to explain the general steps of hypothesis testing. This chapter will prepare you to:

- Describe the purpose for and the process of hypothesis testing
- Correctly state hypotheses
- Distinguish between one-tailed and two-tailed tests of significance
- Describe and distinguish between type I and type II errors
- Describe statistical power and understand its importance in statistical analysis
- Describe effect size and explain its relation to statistical significance
- Understand the differences between statistical and clinical significance
- Understand the place of hypothesis testing in evidence-based practice

Key Terms

Alternative hypothesis

Clinically significant

Effect

Effect size

Generalizability

Null hypothesis

One-tailed test

Statistical power

Two-tailed test

Type I error

Type II error

INTRODUCTION

Let us say that a nurse researcher is interested in studying whether a newly developed intervention for fall prevention is more effective than an existing approach in reducing fall rates. The question is "How do we determine the effect of the new fall prevention intervention compared to an existing one?" We say there is an **effect** when changes in one variable cause another variable to change. Recall that in intervention or experimental studies, the researcher manipulates the independent variable, and then measures change on the dependent variable to determine if an effect is present and the strength of the effect. To determine whether the new intervention has an effect on fall incidence, we need to employ hypothesis testing, which is the process of determining if the observed difference in a variable(s), fall rates in our example, is significant, meaning the likelihood of the observed reduction is not due to chance.

In a more familiar sense, nurses use hypotheses, or informed speculation, routinely in our day-to-day work. We might ask ourselves questions like, "I wonder if Mr. Garcia's low blood pressure is because of a change in medication or fluid volume deficit?" We then collect data that will help us determine the underlying cause of the low blood pressure and take the appropriate measures to manage the problem.

Hypothesis testing in the world of evidence-based practice and research is also about addressing problems, but instead of being directed at decisions for a single patient, we are interested in results that may be applied to the average patient or a target population. Hypothesis testing provides a better understanding of how much confidence we can have in the results—that is, we can estimate the probability that the results are true. In research and evidence-based practice, knowing about the application of results to an average patient or population and our confidence in the results adds up to determine the **generalizability** of results from any given study. Remember that generalizability is the accuracy with which findings from a sample may be applied to the population (due to impracticability of studying an entire population in most occasions). Since a sample is used to make inferences about the population, there will be a chance of making errors. Hypothesis testing is the foundation for making informed decisions about the strength of evidence for practice. There are seven general steps in hypothesis testing, as shown in the following box:

> **General Steps in Hypothesis Testing**
>
> 1. Determine hypotheses.
> 2. Choose the level of significance.
> 3. Propose an appropriate test.
> 4. Check assumptions of the chosen test.
> 5. Compute the test statistics.
> 6. Find the critical value.
> 7. Compare the test statistics and critical value to make conclusions.

GENERAL STEPS IN HYPOTHESIS TESTING

Step 1: Determining Hypotheses

The first step is to set up or state hypotheses; this is an essential part of hypothesis testing. In every study and in many evidence-based practice projects, two hypotheses, the null hypothesis and the alternative hypothesis, are formulated, and they are competing statements.

The hypothesis with no effects is called the **null hypothesis** and is denoted as H_0. The null hypothesis usually is thought of as an objective starting point, or the center of a fulcrum, where there is no statistically discernible difference. For our example, we would write "On average, there is no difference in fall prevention between a newly developed approach and an existing approach." In research and evidence-based practice, we design our studies to test the null hypothesis with the intention of rejecting this hypothesis.

The **alternative hypothesis**, on the other hand, is a hypothesis that states an effect and is denoted as H_1 or H_a; it represents what a researcher really wants to find out. For our example, we may write, "On average, the newly developed approach and an existing approach have a different effect," or "The newly developed approach has a better effect, on average, compared to that of an existing approach for preventing falls."

Step 2: Choosing the Level of Significance

In hypothesis testing, we try to determine whether or not any statistical significance is present that can allow us to better understand the relationship between variables. The level of significance is the criterion used for calculating statistical significance and is determined by a researcher in advance; it has been customary to choose 10% (0.1), 5% (0.05), 1% (0.01), or 0.1% (0.001) for the level of significance. For example, if the researcher is willing to incorrectly reject the null hypothesis 5% of the time, then selecting a level of significance of 0.05 is appropriate.

Step 3: Proposing an Appropriate Test

Once both hypotheses have been formulated, we will determine what statistical test is the best for testing the proposed hypotheses. Each statistical test has requirements in terms of how many variables are being measured and at what level of measurement. Choosing statistical tests is discussed in more detail elsewhere, but **Table 7-1** briefly summarizes key points in selecting an appropriate statistical test.

Choice of research questions, hypotheses, and levels of measurement of variables in those hypotheses are critical in the research process. Let us consider an example null hypothesis: There is no relationship between weight and systolic blood pressure (SBP). We know we are looking into a relationship between two variables, weight and SBP, and both are measured on the ratio level of measurements. This is a perfect hypothesis for using the test statistic, Pearson's correlation coefficient, according to Table 7-1. Note that a nonparametric correlation coefficient such as Spearman's rho should be used if one of the variables is measured on the ordinal level of measurement.

Step 4: Checking Assumptions of the Chosen Test

Once the researcher or clinician knows the category of statistical tests that may be suited for the hypotheses, the assumptions of that test

Table	
7-1	**Choosing a Statistical Test**

Independent Variables (IVs)	Dependent Variable	Statistical Tests
0 IV	Interval & normal	One-sample t-test
	Categorical	χ^2 test of goodness of fit
1 categorical IV with 2 levels (independent)	Interval & normal	Independent t-test
	Ordinal or interval	Wilcoxon/Mann–Whitney test
	Categorical	χ^2/Fisher's exact test
1 categorical IV with 2 levels (dependent)	Interval & normal	Dependent t-test
	Ordinal or interval	Wilcoxon signed rank test
	Categorical	McNemar test
1 categorical IV with more than 2 levels (independent)	Interval & normal	One-way analysis of variance (ANOVA)
	Ordinal or interval	Kruskal–Wallis test
1 categorical IV with more than 2 levels (dependent)	Interval & normal	One-way repeated measures ANOVA
	Ordinal or interval	Friedman test
	Categorical	Repeated measures logistic regression
2 or more categorical IVs (independent)	Interval & normal	Factorial ANOVA
	Categorical	Factorial logistic regression
1 interval IV	Interval & normal	Correlation (Pearson's)/ simple linear regression
	Ordinal or interval	Nonparametric correlation (Spearman's rho)
	Categorical	Simple logistic regression
1 or more interval IVs and/or 1 or more categorical IVs	Interval & normal	Multiple regression/analysis of covariance (ANCOVA)
	Categorical	Logistic regression/ discriminant analysis

must be scrutinized to ensure that the results are trustworthy. Each statistical test, such as Pearson's correlation coefficient, may have unique assumptions, but there are some common assumptions across tests. These include normality (the data values are distributed in a normal curve), equal variance across groups (the variation on each variable in each group is equal), and independence (that there is no overlap of members between groups). The details of these common assumptions will be covered in Chapter 8.

Steps 5 and 6: Running the Proposed Test and Finding the Critical Value

As we proceed in this text, we will discuss each test and how to select the necessary options in SPSS.

Step 7: Comparing Results and Making Conclusions

Hypothesis testing boils down to whether you reject or fail to reject the null hypothesis; that is, is one variable really affecting or influencing another variable or is the result only because of chance? We measure this probability of effect (p) as greater or less than α, where α is the level of significance and where the p-value is the probability that a statistic is significant. When the p-value associated with the test statistics is less than or equal to α, the results are said to be significant, and we reject the null hypothesis in favor of the alternative hypothesis. On the other hand, the results are not significant if the p-value associated with the test statistic is greater than α, and we do not reject the null hypothesis. Figure 7-1 shows the comparison between the p-value and α in reaching a statistical decision.

Hypothesis testing applies to all inferential statistical analyses including hypotheses around associations, examination of differences, prediction, and intervention comparisons. For example, we might be interested in the association between two variables: Is delirium related to the risk for falls? An example of examination of differences is: Are women more likely than men to fall? A hypothesis about prediction of falls might be informally stated, "As the number of medications

Figure 7-1

Comparison between *p*-value and α in reaching a statistical decision.

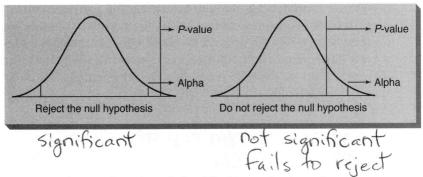

Reject the null hypothesis   Do not reject the null hypothesis

significant   *not significant*
        fails to reject

increases, so does the risk for falls." Hypothesis testing often concerns interventions that are compared; intervention one is more effective than intervention two in preventing falls.

HYPOTHESES

As stated previously, setting up null and alternative hypotheses is the first and most important step of hypothesis testing. These are the two competing statements about your topics of interest. The null hypothesis will always state that there is no expected relationship or difference, while the alternative hypothesis will state there will be an expected relationship or difference.

The null hypothesis gets special attention because the final decision in hypothesis testing is always made with the null hypothesis. At the end of each hypothesis test, a researcher either rejects the null hypothesis or fails to reject the null hypothesis in favor of alternative hypothesis. No one claims to reject or fail to reject the alternative hypothesis! Failing to reject the null hypothesis does not mean that the null hypothesis is true. Rather, it only means that a researcher does not have enough information to reject the null hypothesis in favor of the alternative hypothesis. Rejecting the null hypothesis only suggests that the alternative hypothesis may be true. In this fashion, the results of statistical tests are always discussed tentatively with the understanding that even when the probability of erroneously rejecting the null hypothesis is low, there is always a small chance that such an error has been made. For example, let us say that we have completed hypothesis testing between our two fall prevention approaches and found no statistically significant difference. In our conclusion we might say, "Fall prevention approaches one and two are *likely* to produce the same patient outcomes under similar environmental circumstances." The word, *likely*, makes it clear that there is always a possibility that the findings were observed by chance.

ONE-TAILED VS. TWO-TAILED TESTS OF SIGNIFICANCE

Hypothesis testing can be conducted with either one-tailed or two-tailed tests of significance, depending upon how you set up your hypothesis. Let us consider the previous fall prevention example. Our null hypothesis stated "On average, the number of falls is equal to 13." The alternative hypothesis states, "The number of falls is not equal to 13, on average." We stated these two hypotheses in such a way that shows that we are interested in seeing whether or not there will be a difference between the average number of falls and a known constant of 13, but not specifying whether there would be more or fewer falls (the direction of the difference). This is called a **two-tailed test** because we will look for a significant difference in both directions—greater and fewer falls.

Let us now take into consideration that we are interested in finding the direction of group differences if the results are significant. We may then state our hypotheses in the following manner:

H_0: *The average number of falls is equal to 13.*

H_1: *The average number of falls is less than 13.*

This is called a **one-tailed test** because we will look for a significant difference in one direction only: less than 13. It allows us to estimate the direction of a relationship or group difference, given an expected effect. Hypotheses in tests of significance can be written in different ways, and these are summarized in **Table 7-2**.

Table 7-2	Language for Writing One- and Two-Tailed Hypotheses					
		One-Tailed				
Two-Tailed		**Left-Tailed**		**Right-Tailed**		
Null	**Alternative**	**Null**	**Alternative**	**Null**	**Alternative**	
is	is not	not less than	less than	not greater than	greater than	
equal to	not equal to	at least	less than	at most	greater than	

TYPES OF ERRORS

In hypothesis testing, there are four possible outcomes, including two different types of errors, as shown in **Table 7-3**. A **type I error** occurs when the null hypothesis is rejected by mistake; this error is defined as the probability of rejecting the true null hypothesis. In our fall prevention example, a type I error will occur if we conclude that the newly developed fall prevention approach is more effective than an existing approach when in fact they do not differ.

On the other hand, a **type II error** occurs when the null hypothesis is not rejected when it is actually false. This error is defined as the

Table 7-3	Four Possible Outcomes of a Hypothesis Test	
	Null Hypothesis	
Decision	**True**	**False**
Do not reject null hypothesis	Correct decision	Type II error (β)
Reject null hypothesis	Type I error (α)	Correct decision

probability of not rejecting the false null hypothesis. In our example, a type II error will occur if we conclude that the two fall prevention approaches do not differ in terms of effectiveness when in fact the newly developed approach is more effective.

In general, a type I error is considered to be more serious than a type II error. Consider the implications (cost, training efforts, and new documentation) of implementing a new fall prevention program when it is really not more effective. However, the researcher has some control over type I errors, while the exact probability of a type II error is not known. The researcher chooses the acceptable level of making a type I error before hypothesis testing (setting the α or level of significance) and compares this with the p-values to help to make final conclusions. Essentially, the researcher decides ahead of time what level of type I error he is willing to risk in rejecting the null hypothesis in error: 1 out of 1000 times ($\alpha = 0.001$), 1 out of 100 times ($\alpha = 0.01$), 1 out of 20 times ($\alpha = 0.05$), or 1 out of 10 times ($\alpha = 0.10$).

Type I and type II errors are inversely related in all hypotheses testing, meaning that as the likelihood of making one type of error decreases, the likelihood of making the other type of error increases. If the researcher sets the level of significance too low to decrease the likelihood of making a type I error, the likelihood of making a type II error increases (saying there is no effect when there really is one). However, increasing the sample size is one way of reducing both errors. This makes sense since increasing the sample size will bring the sample closer to the population, which will decrease the chance of committing errors.

TWO-TAILED HYPOTHESIS TESTING WITH AN EXAMPLE

Let us consider an example to explain how hypothesis testing is done. We will perform a two-tailed test in which we suspect that the average number of falls is not equal to 13. We will take a sample of 40 participants to test the claim and assume that the population standard deviation, sigma (σ), is known as 4.

Step 1: Determine Hypotheses

The two competing hypotheses are:

H_0: *The average number of falls is equal to 13.*
H_1: *The average number of falls is not equal to 13.*

or

$$H_0: \mu = 13$$
$$H_1: \mu \neq 13$$

where μ is the average number of falls.

Step 2: Choose the Level of Significance

The next step is to choose the level of significance, or alpha (α). This is essentially the same as the type I error and specifies how confident you want to be in rejecting the null hypothesis. If you have chosen a type I error of 0.05, for example, it means that you are comfortable in making errors up to 5 times in 100 hypothesis tests. We will use an α of 0.05 for this example.

Step 3: Propose an Appropriate Test

In the current step, we are to propose a statistical test that will help us make the decision to reject or not to reject the null hypothesis. In this case, we are comparing a group average against a single known average, and a one-sample z test will be the appropriate test.

Step 4: Check Assumptions of the Chosen Test

Before we conduct a proposed test, we need to check assumptions required by the proposed test, a one-sample z test. The test requires that a sample size is large enough and the population standard deviation is known. In this example, our sample size is 40 and it is large enough. In addition, the population standard deviation is known to be 4. The last assumption to be met is that the sampling distribution of the sample mean will be approximately normally distributed and we will assume that this has been met.

Step 5: Run the Proposed Test

We then compute the test statistic, and the test statistic formula for a one-sample z test is

$$Z = \frac{\bar{x} - \mu}{\frac{\sigma}{\sqrt{n}}}$$

where $\bar{x}$ is the sample mean, μ is the population mean, σ is the known population standard deviation, and n is the sample size. So, the test statistics for our example will be

$$Z = \frac{\bar{x} - \mu}{\frac{\sigma}{\sqrt{n}}} = \frac{11 - 13}{\frac{4}{\sqrt{40}}} = -3.16$$

based on data showing that the average number of falls for the 40 participants was 11.

Step 6: Find Critical Values

Next, you must find the critical value, which depends upon your chosen level of significance, alpha. We chose 0.05 for our level of significance earlier, and we are performing a two-tailed test of significance, as we are interested only in whether or not there is a difference between the two approaches. Therefore, we get two rejection regions on both tails of the normal distribution with the corresponding probabilities

of $\frac{\alpha}{2} = 0.025$, as shown in **Figure 7-2**, and the corresponding critical values are -1.96 and $+1.96$.

Figure 7-2

Rejection region of the two-tailed test of significance.

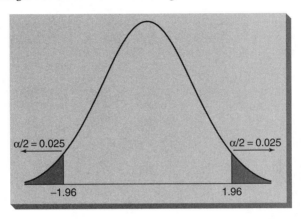

Step 7: Compare Results and Make Conclusions

In the final step, we compare the test statistics and critical values and make conclusions about our hypotheses. Our computed test statistic was −3.16, and this falls within one of the rejection regions, as it is smaller than the critical value, −1.96, as shown in **Figure 7-3**.

Figure 7-3

Making decisions in hypothesis testing.

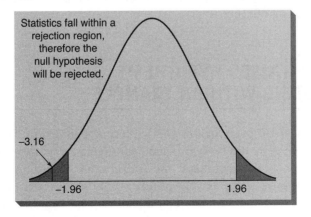

Figure 7-4

Decision making with *p*-value and the level of significance.

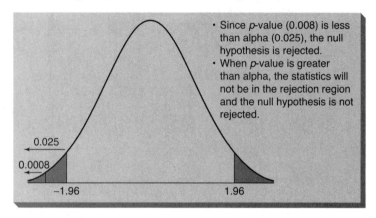

- Since *p*-value (0.008) is less than alpha (0.025), the null hypothesis is rejected.
- When *p*-value is greater than alpha, the statistics will not be in the rejection region and the null hypothesis is not rejected.

0.025

0.0008

−1.96   1.96

Therefore, our decision is to reject the null hypothesis. We conclude that the average number of falls is not equal to 13.

We can obtain the same results by comparing the level of significance with the *p*-value, which depends upon the computed statistics. The *p*-value is, by definition, the probability that a statistic becomes significant. When the *p*-value is less than the chosen level of significance, we reject the null hypothesis as the result is unlikely. On the other hand, the null hypothesis will not be rejected if the *p*-value is greater than the chosen level of significance. **Figure 7-4** summarizes the decision making through the comparison of the *p*-value and the level of significance.

ONE-TAILED HYPOTHESIS TESTING WITH AN EXAMPLE

If we were to perform a one-tailed test of significance for the same example as we did for two-tailed hypothesis, everything will stay the same except the hypotheses and critical value. With a one-tailed test, we suspect that the average number of falls is less than 13. We will still assume that we know that the average fall rate with an existing intervention is 13 falls in a sample of 40 participants. We will use $\sigma = 4$ for our fall prevention example. Our hypotheses now reflect direction.

H_0: *The average number of falls is equal to 13.*
H_1: *The average number of falls is less than 13.*

or

$$H_0: \mu = 13$$
$$H_1: \mu < 13$$

where μ is the average number of falls. We will use the same level of significance of 0.05 for a one-tailed, one-sample z test.

Our sample test statistics is the same as before:

$$Z = \frac{\bar{x} - \mu}{\frac{\sigma}{\sqrt{n}}} = \frac{11 - 13}{\frac{4}{\sqrt{40}}} = -3.16$$

but our critical value will change. With a proposed one-tailed test, we will get only one rejection region on left tail of the normal distribution, as shown in **Figure 7-5**, and the corresponding critical value is -1.645.

Figure 7-5

Rejection region of the one-tailed test of significance.

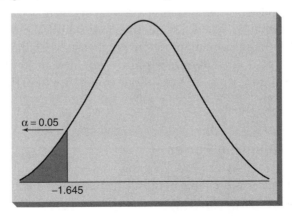

Figure 7-6

Making decisions in hypothesis testing.

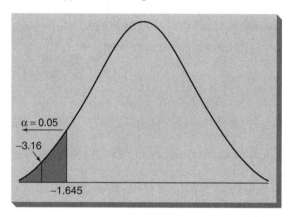

Our computed test statistic of -3.16 falls within the rejection region as it is smaller than the critical value, -1.645, as shown in **Figure 7-6**. Therefore, our decision is to reject the null hypothesis and conclude that the average number of falls is less than 13.

STATISTICAL POWER

Statistical power is the probability of rejecting the null hypothesis when it is false, or of correctly saying there is an effect when it exists. Remember that a type II error (β) is the probability of not rejecting a null hypothesis when it is false, or of saying there is no difference in effect when there actually is one. Therefore, statistical power is equal to $1 - \beta$. From this equation, we can see that statistical power increases as the type II error decreases and we would want to obtain higher statistical power for the sake of our confidence in making the right conclusions.

Factors Influencing Power

Higher power is desirable in most situations, and there are a number of factors that can influence statistical power, including the level of significance, effect size, sample size, and the type of statistical test. The level of significance is the designated probability of making a type I error, and this is a criterion used for determining statistical significance when the null hypothesis is true. For example, the probability of observing the difference between the average number of falls and a constant of 13 when the null hypothesis is true should be less than 0.01 to be significant if the level of significance of 0.01 was chosen. In general, you will obtain the greatest statistical power when you increase the level of significance, since type I error and type II error are in an inverse relationship and the power is $1 - \beta$.

Effect size is the magnitude of the relationship or difference found in a hypothesis test. When hypothesis testing indicates that a relationship or difference is statistically significant, it does not tells us how big the effect, relationship, or difference is—all that statistical significance says is that there is a relationship or difference. For example, the statistically significant result we found with our two-tailed fall prevention example only tells us that the average number of falls is less than 13; it does not calculate the magnitude of the difference between the approaches. However, the effect size tells us the clinical importance of a statistically significant finding. In general, the statistical power increases as the effect size increases. More details about effect size are covered in the next section.

Statistical power also increases as the sample size increases. When the sample size is small, our chance of accurately representing the population is lower and the results may not be generalizable. Therefore, the probability of making the correct decision to reject or not reject the null hypothesis is lower. The larger the sample, the more likely the sample will represent the population and the higher the probability of making the correct decision.

The last factor, the type of statistical test, will also influence the probability of rejecting the null hypothesis. In general, a larger sample size is required when you choose more complex statistical tests.

Types of Power Analysis

Power analyses are performed to determine what elements are needed to reject the null hypothesis when it should be rejected. You can conduct power analysis before or after the study is completed.

When conducted before the study is completed, it is called an a priori power analysis, and it is a guide for estimating the sample size required to detect statistical significance and correctly reject the null hypothesis. On the other hand, if you conduct a power analysis after the study is completed, it is called a post hoc power analysis and tells you what level of power the study was conducted at with the obtained sample size, along with other factors. While post hoc analyses are an option, researchers usually conduct an a priori power analysis. Most researchers take the minimum power of 0.80 as acceptable for their tests (i.e., there should be less than 20% chance of committing a type II error).

Meanings and Interpretations

Statistical power is the probability of rejecting a false null hypothesis and is stated as a probability between 0 and 1. In other words, statistical power tells us how often we can correctly reject a null hypothesis and say there is a true effect. In interpreting the results of any study, how much power the study had in detecting an effect if the effect exists should be carefully considered.

Suppose a clinician wanted to determine whether ownership of hospitals (private vs. public) is related to the frequency of surgical mistakes. The researcher recruited a sample size of 104 to obtain 80% power, suggested by an a priori power analysis. If there is an actual difference in the numbers of surgical mistakes between public and private hospitals, it implies that this study will observe statistically significant results in 80% of studies and nonstatistically significant results in the other 20% of studies.

Results from a study without enough power should be interpreted with caution, and additional studies with larger sample sizes to increase the statistical power will be required before concluding that there was an effect.

EFFECT SIZE

Platts-Mills and colleagues (2012) found that emergency providers reported lower satisfaction regarding access to information for residents from skilled nursing facilities (SNF) that accept Medicaid (7.13 versus

8.15, $p < 0.001$) versus those that did not. Based on these findings, should SNF make absolute statements that facilities should not accept Medicaid so that emergency providers are more satisfied with access to necessary information and provide better services? No! Even if the same variables are being studied, one study may obtain a statistically significant result while the other study may not, depending upon numerous factors such as how the sample was obtained, the size of the sample, and the research settings. Statistical significance alone does not tell us much about how much of an effect was present and how important the size of effect is in practice.

Many researchers report whether or not an intervention or relationship between variables of interest was statistically significant, but not the magnitude of the effect of interest in the study. The measure of the strength or magnitude of an effect, difference, or relationship between variables is effect size, and it helps us to evaluate the clinical importance of the study given a statistical significance. Effect size may be thought of as a dose-response curve or rate. We are often exposed to this idea when evaluating how an individual patient responds to medication therapy; that is, different doses of a drug have differing magnitudes of effect. Aspirin prescribed at 80 mg daily has little analgesic effect, but when increased to 650 mg, aspirin has an analgesic effect that is noticeable. We understand that the **effect** of aspirin differs with the dose. We can measure similar effects of other interventions, including our fall prevention approach. An intervention with a large effect size is more likely to produce the clinical effect that we are looking for. Therefore, effect size allows us to make a more meaningful inference from a sample to a population.

Types of Effect Size

There are several measures of effect size, including Cohen's d, Pearson's r coefficient, ω^2, and others. However, we will only discuss Cohen's d and Pearson's r, as these two measures are most commonly used.

Cohen's d is simply the difference of the two population means divided by the standard deviation of the data and is shown in the following formula:

$$d = \frac{\overline{x_1} - \overline{x_2}}{s}$$

where s is the standard deviation of either group when the variances of the two groups are equal, or

$$s = \sqrt{\frac{(n_1 - 1)s_1^2 + (n_2 - 1)s_2^2}{n_1 + n_2}}$$

when the variances of the two groups are not equal. For hypothesis testing, you will get a statistically significant result when the two samples means are very different from each other. When this is the case, Cohen's d will be large, indicating that there is a large effect size; effect size is small if the value of Cohen's d is around 0.2, medium if the value is around 0.5, and large if the value is around 0.8 (Cohen, 1988). Note that the use of Cohen's definition for small, medium, and large effect size can be misleading. For example, Cohen's d of 0.8 indicates a large effect size, but this effect size may not be clinically important.

Pearson's r coefficient allows an examination of the relationship between two variables. It is the easiest coefficient to compute and interpret, and it can be calculated from many statistics. For example, Pearson's r coefficient as an effect size can be found by the following equation:

$$r = \sqrt{\frac{t^2}{t^2 + df}}$$

where t is the t-test statistic and df is the degrees of freedom. Details of these two statistics will be discussed in Chapter 11. The value varies between -1 and $+1$, and the effect size is small if the value varies around 0.1, medium if the value varies around 0.3, and large if the value varies around 0.5.

Meanings and Interpretation

Effect sizes are important because they are an objective measure of how large an effect was in a study, regardless of study setting, and they allow the nurse to consider the practical/clinical importance through the magnitude of the effect in addition to the statistical significance.

It is possible that a statistically significant result may not be practically or **clinically significant**, and a statistically nonsignificant result may be practically or clinically significant. For example, a study may have had a statistically nonsignificant result due to small sample size, yet demonstrate a large effect size of a newly developed medicine to treat HIV. Or, a study may have had a statistically significant result due to an excessively large sample size, yet have such a small effect size that application to individual patients is not possible. The practical/clinical importance of the study should be determined with careful consideration about the sample size and the nature of the study being conducted.

SUMMARY

Hypothesis testing allows researchers and clinicians to make informed decisions about the nature of study results by incorporating probability of the decision being true into the decision-making process. Hypothesis testing involves seven general steps: (1) determining hypotheses, (2) choosing the level of significance, (3) proposing an appropriate test, (4) checking assumptions of the chosen test, (5) computing the test statistics, (6) finding the critical value, and (7) comparing the test statistics and critical value to make decisions and conclusions.

Two hypotheses, the null and alternative hypotheses, are formulated, and they are two competing statements. The hypothesis with no effects is called the null hypothesis, denoted as H_0, and the hypothesis with an effect is called the alternative hypothesis, denoted as H_1 or H_a.

Level of significance (α) is normally chosen from among 0.01, 0.05, and 0.10, and the corresponding statistical test should be carefully chosen to reflect level of measurement and number of variables.

Hypothesis testing can be either a one-tailed or two-tailed test of significance. Two-tailed tests of significance determine only whether or not there is an effect, while one-tailed tests also determine the direction of an effect.

Since a sample is used to make inferences about the population, there will be a chance of making errors. Two types of error in hypothesis testing are type I error and type II error. A type I error is the probability of rejecting a true null hypothesis, and a type II error is the probability of not rejecting a false null hypothesis. The researcher can influence error making by selecting an alpha level and sample size.

Statistical power is the probability of rejecting a null hypothesis when it is false and equal to $1 - \beta$. Factors such as the level of significance, effect size, sample size, and the type of statistical test affect statistical power. A power analysis helps in determining sample size and the power of specific statistical tests, given sample size.

Effect size is the measure of strength for an effect, difference, or relationship between variables and helps us to evaluate how much an effect was present, given a statistical significance. It allows us to evaluate the practical or clinical significance of an effect with an objective measure, separately from the statistical significance.

Critical Thinking Questions

1. What will happen to the statistical power if the sample size increases? Explain.
2. Suppose you rejected a null hypothesis at 1% level of significance. Would you reject the same null hypothesis at 5% level? Explain.
3. Suppose you rejected a null hypothesis at 5% level of significance. Does this mean that you would get the same level of statistical significance if you were to do the experiment over multiple times? Explain.
4. What is the difference between statistical significance and clinical significance?

Self-Quiz www

1. A type I error is made when:
   a. the false null hypothesis is not rejected.
   b. the true alternative hypothesis is rejected.
   c. the true null hypothesis is rejected.
   d. the false alternative hypothesis is not rejected.
2. A null hypothesis was rejected at the 1% level, and the results were determined to be statistically significant. What would this mean?
   a. The null hypothesis is absolutely wrong.
   b. The null hypothesis is probably wrong. *may be true*
   c. The alternative hypothesis is right. —
   d. None of the above

3. True or false: A medical researcher recently developed a new medicine and wants to test its effectiveness. He collected a sample of 80 patients, divided them into a control and experimental group, and performed an experiment. The experiment showed the average difference in treating time was significant between the control and experimental groups at 0.05 levels and Cohen's *d* came out to be 0.06. Since the effect size was very small, he should discard his study results.

REFERENCES

Cohen, J. (1988). *Statistical power analysis for the behavioral sciences* (2nd ed.). Hillsdale, NJ: Erlbaum.

Platts-Mills, T. F., Biese, K., LaMantia, M., Zamora, Z., Patel, L. N., McCall, B., … Kizer, J. S. (2012). Nursing home revenue source and information availability during the emergency department evaluation of nursing home residents. *Journal of the American Medical Directors Association, 13*(4), 332–336.

Chapter

8 Getting Ready for the Analysis

Learning Objectives

The principal goal of this chapter is to explain the importance of checking the quality of collected data and the assumptions of the proposed tests. This chapter will prepare you to:

- Define missing data and outliers and understand how they can affect an analysis negatively
- Understand possible remedies for missing data and outliers
- Understand the importance of checking assumptions of statistical tests prior to analysis

Key Terms

Data cleaning

Nonrandom missing
  data

Outlier

Random missing data

Skewed

INTRODUCTION

Elsewhere, we have discussed the general steps of conducting hypothesis testing. Before proceeding to conduct hypothesis testing, however, the researcher must ensure that data are clean and free of any errors. **Data cleaning** is an important first step in every data analysis. Any erroneous data should be corrected before the analysis to prevent the introduction of error in the results. Data cleaning should be done in the early stages of the study.

Let us consider, for example, the variable "citizenship." We have specified "citizen" and "noncitizen" and would expect to have only two possible responses. If another variable, "age," is considered, we would expect to see the measurements only within certain limits; if we are studying adults between the ages of 18 and 24, then the responses on that variable should be between those limits. For both citizenship and age, we would be concerned if a response is missing or if a variable has a value outside the expected range. If the data are not accurate, the inferred results will not be accurate either.

Errors can be introduced into data and results via missing data, outliers, violation of the assumptions for the proposed statistical tests, incorrect data entry, and data loss. Errors in data are part of every study, and a responsible researcher should have a plan for managing them in order to make accurate statements about statistical results. For nurses engaged in evidence-based practice, it is important to scrutinize reports of research to identify how errors have been treated in the analysis, which is a criterion for determining the quality of the findings. Errors are a threat to both internal and external validity of a study—for example, large amounts of missing data may limit either conclusions about the effect of an independent variable on the dependent variable or the generalizability of study findings.

MISSING DATA

Missing data occurs when a research participant or subject fails to provide responses to a variable, when data are inadvertently left out, or when a researcher has not found a way of measuring a variable. There are several ways of dealing with missing data, and how serious a problem it poses depends on the amount, as well as the pattern, of missing data (i.e., whether the data are missing at random or nonrandom). Sometimes the problem is simply one of transcription, with the person entering data having mistakenly omitted some value or set of values. Transcription errors are easily corrected by returning to the original data and making the necessary changes in the statistical software database.

Random vs. Nonrandom Missing

The pattern of missing data has to do with whether the data are missing randomly or nonrandomly; this is often times a more important issue than how much of the data set is missing. Understanding why and how the data are missing can help greatly in finding the correct solution.

Random Pattern of Missing Data

Missing data is considered random when it is scattered in the database without any pattern. For example, let us assume that a study was done about the relationship between income and health. If some participants across different income levels did not provide information on their health, the missing data on health is not related to the level of income; this is considered to be **random missing data**.

Nonrandom Pattern of Missing Data

On the other hand, missing data is considered nonrandom when a specific pattern in the database is apparent. **Nonrandom missing data** are more problematic, since the pattern will distort the results and jeopardize internal and external validity. For example, consider a situation where a researcher is conducting a study to investigate the relationship between gender and smoking. If the women consistently do not provide information on their smoking habits, but most of the men do, then the missing data on smoking is related to gender and the data are said to be nonrandom missing. In this example, the researcher will not be able to report with any confidence on the relationship between smoking and gender.

The pattern of missing data is important, but the volume of missing data can also be problematic. In general, the problem gets worse as the amount of missing data increases. There is no black and white answer for how much missing data can be tolerated; the researcher must judge the effect of data loss on statistical power.

Remedies for Missing Data

Missing data is a serious problem in data analysis as it can affect the generalizability of the results, and so it needs careful handling. There are several potential remedies to missing data. The decision of how to handle missing data is crucial and should be made in the context of the given problem.

Deletion

The simplest approach to deal with missing data is to delete those cases with missing data and then run the data analyses with only the complete cases. However, this approach only works if there is little missing data and if the missing data are random. If there is a large number of missing data in comparison to the total sample size, deleting those cases will result in a substantial loss of information. In addition, there could be a serious distortion of the data if the missing data is not random. The rule of thumb is to delete the missing data only if a small amount of the data is missing, say 5% or less, and it is in a random pattern.

Estimation

The next approach is to estimate the missing values and use these in the data analysis. Estimation still introduces bias into the analysis but is useful when the sample size is small and the deletion of missing data will create further problems. There are several popular estimation procedures to replace missing data, such as utilizing prior knowledge, substituting with mean values, estimating with regression models, expectation maximization, and multiple imputations. We will discuss the most straightforward approaches: utilizing prior knowledge and substituting with mean values.

Using prior knowledge may be the simplest estimation approach, as it uses a well-educated guess from prior knowledge to substitute for the missing data. This is an adequate estimation procedure if you have extensive experience with a research area and when the sample size is small. For example, a nurse carrying out a quality improvement project is collecting data on the ratio of nurses to patients in the general medical units. The nurse, having worked on these units for some years and having conducted similar projects, knows that the range is from 1:4 on the day shift to 1:6 on the night shift. When encountering missing data from a few shifts, the nurse substitutes these values on the basis of experience.

Substituting missing data with mean values is another simple approach for estimating missing data. In this case, the researcher calculates an arithmetic average or mean from the available data, and that mean is used to replace the missing data. This approach is convenient because a calculated mean replaces each missing data point and it often provides a more accurate estimation than prior knowledge. A quick example would be to replace missing data on average daily number of medication errors with an average from the previous month. However, this estimation approach reduces the variability in the data set, as the mean value replacing the missing data will always differ from the original missing values. If the data is divided by a grouping variable, the mean values should be computed for the groups, separately.

OUTLIERS

Any data value that is not a common or expected value for a variable of measurement is considered an **outlier**. For example, in our study of adults between the ages of 18 and 24, perhaps all but one participant are 18–20 years old. The one participant who is 24 years old is an outlier relative to the younger members of the study. Consider an example scatterplot, shown in **Figure 8-1**.

You will see that the scatterplot shows that the data points are relatively close to each other from the center. However, the center line of

Figure 8-1

Example scatterplot for weight and systolic blood pressure.

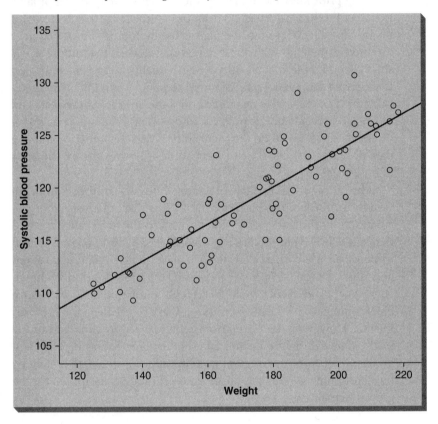

this plot is shifted upward (as shown in **Figure 8-2**) when a data value in the upper right-hand portion of the scatterplot is introduced. This is because the unusually large data value has increased the probable mean value. Since outliers can introduce errors in the analysis, special attention is required to identify and handle them.

Spotting the Outliers

Sometimes it may be difficult to determine whether an observation or measurement is an outlier, and the decision can be somewhat

Figure 8-2

Scatterplot for weight and systolic blood pressure with an outlier.

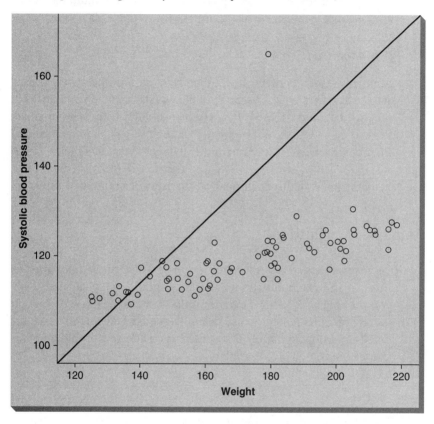

subjective. However, the following are commonly used approaches in identifying the outlier in a data set.

Visual Check Using Graphs and Plots

A review of visual displays of data, such as graphs and plots, is the easiest way of identifying outliers. Observations or data points that are far away from the mass of data should be considered outliers. Two graphical displays useful for identifying the outliers are the *scatterplot* and *box plot*. You should be able to easily identify the outliers as we saw in the scatterplots in Figure 8-1 and Figure 8-2. Box plots are also useful in identifying outliers; any data values that are either below the lower whisker or above the upper whisker are identified as outliers. You will recall from Chapter 5, that the lower whisker equals 1.5 times the minimum data value and the upper whisker equals 1.5 times the maximum data value.

Using Standardized Scores

Another way of identifying the outliers is to examine the corresponding standardized score (i.e., z-scores) of the raw data. When you transform the raw data into z-scores, if the z-scores are unusually large or small, those data values should be treated as the outliers. A general rule of thumb is that a data value is an outlier if its corresponding z-score is outside of the −3 to +3 range, as we would expect 99.8% of all data values in the set to fall in this range per characteristics of a normal distribution.

Remedies for Outliers

Because outliers are a serious problem in data analysis and can threaten internal and external validity, remedies should be considered. First, you should check to see if a transcription error is the cause of the outlier. If not, other remedies may be implemented. Like missing data, the decision of how to handle the outliers is crucial and should be made in the context of a given problem.

Deletion

The simplest way to deal with outliers is to delete those cases that are unusual and then run the data analysis with normal cases. However, this approach should be considered only if there is strong evidence that the unusual data value is not a part of the intended population for the study and the number of outliers is small. For example, you know that a person who is 25 years old is not a part of your population if you defined your intended population as people who are older than 50 years old.

Transform the Data

When outliers are present in the data set, the distribution of the data will likely be **skewed**. Please refer to Chapter 6 for the detailed discussion on skewness. The outlier is pulling the mean of the data in one direction or another, and this will lead to a violation of the commonly required assumption of normality (i.e., normal distribution of the variable). Transformation (arithmetic manipulation) of the data may seem to distort the data, but since all data values are transformed, the consistency between values remains the same and the relationship in the data values still stays the same. There are four commonly used transformation approaches: log transformation, square root transformation, reciprocal transformation, and reverse transformation. The first three transformation approaches attempt to correct problems with positive skewness and the reverse transformation attempts to correct problems with negative skewness. Among approaches for correcting positive skewness, log transformation is for mild skewness, square root transformation is for moderate skewness, and reciprocal transformation is for severe skewness. If you are unsure how severe the skewness problem is, the best approach may be to do trial and error and to see which one transforms the distribution to normal.

Each transformation approach can be performed in SPSS using "Compute Variable" under the Transform pull-down menu. In the "Compute Variable" dialogue box, as shown in **Figure 8-3**, you give a target variable a name and write a transformation function you would

Figure 8-3

The Compute Variable dialogue box in SPSS.

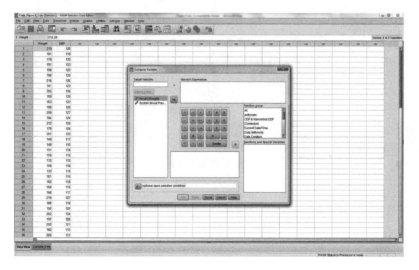

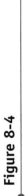

Figure 8-4

Example histograms of transformed variable, systolic blood pressure.

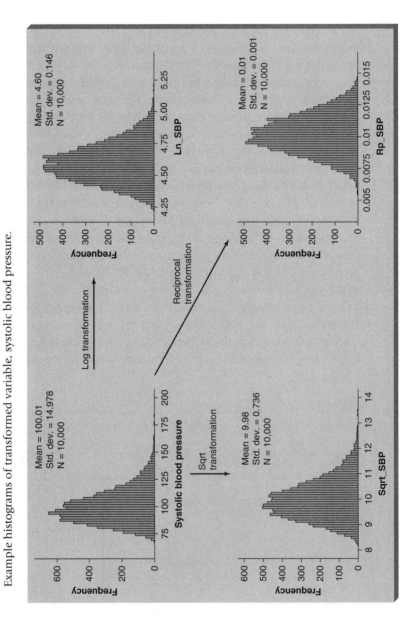

like to perform under the "Numeric Expression" subwindow. It is important to then check whether or not the transformation corrected the problem with the outliers; histograms can be used for this purpose, and an example of how to decide which transformation is the most appropriate is shown in **Figure 8-4**. In this example, the reciprocal transformation of the original variable, SBP, seems to correct the issue of skewness the best.

Changing the Score

If transforming the data fails to correct the problems associated with outliers, you can consider changing the data value(s). However, this approach should be taken as the last resort, as it can seem unethical to manipulate the original data value. To minimize this, the changed score is still treated as an outlier, but has diminished biasing effect on the data analysis results. Changing the score can be done by one of the following methods:

1. Changing the data value to one unit above the largest data value, excluding the outlier. Let us assume, for example, that a researcher is using a 200-point scale and has three outliers of 189, 192, and 199. If the next largest score other than these three outliers is 142, the researcher may change these values to 143.
2. Converting any data with a z-score of 3.29 or larger back to the original data scale using $x = z \times s + \mu$, where x is the converted data value, z is the z-score, s is the standard deviation, and μ is the mean. This value is chosen since a z-score of 3.28 is often considered as an outlier. In this example, we have reduced the effect of the outliers 189, 192, and 199 by converting to a score of 149.48 while they still remain as outliers.

ASSUMPTIONS OF PARAMETRIC TESTS

Most of the statistical tests being described in this text are types of *parametric tests*. These tests require that certain assumptions are met; if these assumptions are not met, the statistical results will not be accurate. Therefore, it is important to check whether the required assumptions are met before conducting the proposed analysis.

The assumptions for parametric tests are as follows.

1. *Data should be normally distributed*. You may think that this assumption is easy to check. However, you should be careful with this assumption, because what has to be normally distributed may differ for different statistical tests. It may be the dependent variable for some tests, while for others it may be the error values that have to be normally distributed. Brief comments about normality distribution will be made elsewhere. The normality assumption can be checked in several ways. First, it can be checked visually through histograms or P-P plots. In a histogram, you will want to see a symmetrical bell-curved distribution if the data are normally distributed. A P-P plot is the cumulative probability distribution of a variable against the cumulative probability normal distribution. You would want to see the majority of data values fall on or close to the upward of the right diagonal line. If the data values deviate much from this diagonal line, the data distribution is said to be nonnormal. An example P-P plot is shown in **Figure 8-5**. Second, you can use the measures of skewness and kurtosis. These measures should fall in the -1 to $+1$ range if the data are normal. Lastly, you can perform statistical tests: the Kolomogorov–Smirnov test and/or the Shapiro–Wilk test. To perform these tests, go to Analyze > Descriptive Statistics > Explore in SPSS. Click the Statistics button and then check "Normality plots with tests." When the p-value associated with both tests is less than alpha, the test is determined to be significant and the assumption is said to be violated. If not, you are okay with the normality assumption. An example output is shown in **Table 8-1**.

2. *Data should be measured at interval or ratio level.*

3. *Independence of the data.* As with determining if data are normally distributed, you should be careful with this assumption because different statistical tests require different data to be independent. This assumption has to do with errors that are uncorrelated if the proposed statistical tests are the type of regression analysis. Durbin–Watson statistics is an example of testing this assumption and will be discussed in Chapter 10. However, when the proposed statistical tests are to compare groups, this assumption means that the individuals in different groups have to be independent from each other for group comparison tests.

Figure 8-5

Example P-P plot.

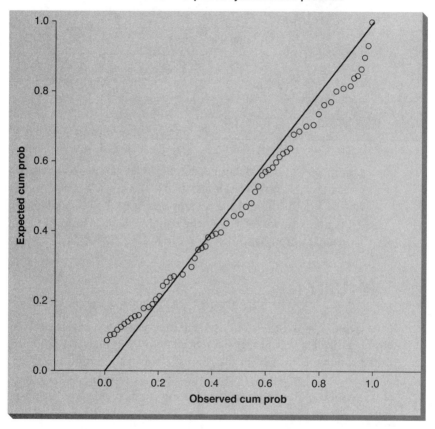

Normal P-P plot of systolic blood pressure

This case is relatively straightforward to examine and will be discussed in Chapter 11.

4. *Equality of variance.* This assumption states that the variance should be equal. If the proposed test is to compare groups, this assumption means that the variance across groups should be equal. If the proposed test is to examine a relationship, this assumption means that the variance of one variable should be equal at all levels of the other variables. Levene's test is one of several tests used for testing this assumption and will be

Table	
8-1	**Example Outputs of Statistical Tests for Normality**

	Tests of Normality					
	Kolmogorov–Smirnov[a]			Shapiro–Wilk		
	Statistic	df	Sig.	Statistic	df	Sig.
Systolic blood pressure	.104	76	.040	.774	76	.000

[a]Lilliefors significance correction

discussed in more detail in Chapter 11. When the *p*-value associated with Levene's test is less than alpha, the test is determined to be significant and the assumption is said to be violated. If it is not, you are okay with the equal variance assumption. An example output is shown in **Table 8-2**.

SUMMARY

Data cleaning is an important first step for every data analysis, and any errors in the data set should be corrected before the analysis to prohibit the introduction of error in the results. Errors can be introduced into data and results in various ways, including via missing data, outliers, and violation of the necessary assumptions to be met for the proposed statistical tests.

Table	
8-2	**Example Output of Levene's Test Results**

	Test of Homogeneity of Variances			
	Levene Statistic	df1	df2	Sig.
Systolic blood pressure	.033	1	74	.856

Missing data occurs when a subject does not provide responses to a variable, data are skipped in data entry, or when a researcher found no way of measuring a variable. We need to pay careful attention to the pattern of missing data, as nonrandom missing data is a more serious problem than random missing data. In general, the problem gets worse as the amount of missing data increases. Missing data can be handled through either deletion or estimation. Deletion should be done only if the amount of missing data is small and it is missing in a random pattern. Otherwise, missing data should be estimated.

Outliers are another important source of errors in data and are defined as any unusual data value in the data set. Outliers can be spotted through visual displays like scatterplots or by transforming the raw data into z-scores. Outliers can be handled through deletion, transformation, or changing the score. Deletion should be done only if you have a sound reason to do so; otherwise transformation should be performed. If transformation does not solve the problem, you should consider changing the score.

All parametric tests require some assumptions to be met. Common assumptions include normality of the data, independence of the data, interval data, and the equality of variance. These assumptions should be checked before the data analysis is performed, as violations of the assumptions can distort the results.

Critical Thinking Questions www

1. Why should the researcher examine the data before conducting data analysis? Explain.
2. Where would information about the treatment of missing data be found in a report of research?
3. Suppose that one of the collected variables was "Birth Year" and we found out that one of the respondents wrote down the current year instead of his actual year of birth. What seems to be an appropriate action for this data?
4. Use the data file called *satisfaction.sav* (found on the Student Companion Website using the access code card from the front of this text), and see which transformation method seems the most reasonable approach with an outlier(s).

Self-Quiz www.

1. True or false: Normality is assumed with all parametric statistical tests; therefore, it is important to check whether the collected data is normally distributed.
2. True or false: Suppose that some female respondents decided not to answer on the question for weight. This type of missing data is considered as random missing.

9 Examining Relationships Between and Among Variables

Learning Objectives

The principal goal of this chapter is to explain how the relationships between variables can be statistically expressed and to discover how the relationship coefficients should be interpreted. This chapter will prepare you to:

- Explain the concepts of correlation and compute the necessary values to analyze data
- Evaluate the assumptions of correlation analyses
- Understand different measures of correlation and choose the appropriate one
- Report the necessary findings in correct APA style
- Understand the purpose of correlational analyses in evidence-based practice

Key Terms www

Association	Correlation
Causality	Covariance
Coefficient of determination	Partial correlation coefficient

INTRODUCTION

"Our analyses suggest a very strong relationship between the numbers of physicians' visits and the rate of 30-day skilled nursing facility re-hospitalization" (Mor, Intrator, Feng, & Grabowski, 2010, p. 62). Like these researchers, we are often interested in investigating a relationship between and/or among variables.

Let us consider an example where researchers examined the relationship between the numbers of cigarettes smoked and the probability of getting lung cancer. We would expect that the probability of getting lung cancer would increase as the numbers of cigarettes smoked increases. When the relationship between two variables moves in the same direction (as one increases, so does the other), the variables are said to be *positively related*. Conversely, if the relationship between variables moves in the opposite direction (such as when the number of medical errors goes up, patient satisfaction declines), the variables are said to be *negatively related*. There may be no relationship between variables if they do not seem to show either positive or negative patterns. For example, we would say that there is no **association** between income and number of wellness visits if the income level is not correlated with an increase or decrease in the number of visits to a health professional for a regular check-up.

In this text, we will discuss how to examine a relationship between and/or among variables, how to interpret visual displays of the relationships, how to choose from the different types of correlation coefficients, and how to interpret these to determine the relationship.

Case Study

Burtson, P. L., & Stichler, J. F. (2010). Nursing work environment and nurse caring: Relationship among motivational factors. *Journal of Advanced Nursing, 66*(8), 1819–1831. doi: 0.1111/j.1365-2648.2010.05336.x

In 2010, Paige L. Burtson and Jaynelle F. Stichler published a study in the *Journal of Advanced Nursing* examining the relationships between variables in the nursing work environment and nurse caring. They used a cross-sectional correlational research design and tested their hypotheses using Pearson's *r*, a correlation coefficient. Burtson and Stichler speculated that factors such as burnout and compassion might be related to nurse caring and noted that the literature supports a relationship between caring from nurses and patient satisfaction. By exploring these relationships, they hoped to shed light on those practices that promote caring and patient satisfaction. Their hypotheses included:

- Hypotheses 1 and 2: Compassion satisfaction (H1) and nurse job satisfaction (H2) are positively correlated with nurse caring.
- Hypotheses 3, 4, and 5: Stress (H3), burnout (H4), and compassion fatigue (H5) are negatively correlated with nurse caring.

Burtson and Stichler analyzed results from a convenience sample of 450 nurses from a single hospital and rejected the null hypotheses in all cases, calculating Pearson's *r* coefficients ranging from ± 0.10 to 0.51 with *p*-values ranging from .05 to .001. Their findings confirmed that as compassion satisfaction and job satisfaction rose, so did nurse caring, indicating a positive relationship between these variables. On the other hand, as stress, burnout, and compassion fatigue rose, nurse caring declined, indicating a negative correlation.

What does a correlational study like the Burtson and Stichler article tell us? How can we use it in practice or as a basis for other research? Correlational studies tell us whether or not a statistically significant relationship exists between variables and the direction of that relationship. Correlational studies are considered exploratory in nature, shedding light on how variables might be connected and whether or not one variable may predict another. When no other research is available, correlational studies may provide insight into human behavior and allow us to consider those variables in our practice. In the preceding case study, as nurse burnout increased, nurse caring decreased. It makes sense in the context of other research and theory to suggest that nurses who are burned out may behave in a less caring manner. We can make policies and consider changing practice if the correlational evidence is consistent from study to study.

Correlational research often provides a foundation for designing and testing interventions—that is, once we know that one variable (burnout) may influence another variable (nurse caring), we can design an experimental study to determine if there is a cause-and-effect relationship. Experimental studies include controlling and manipulating the independent variable (nurse burnout) to determine the effect on the dependent variable (nurse caring). Only experimental studies allow us to determine cause (burnout) and effect (nurse caring).

MEASURING RELATIONSHIPS

Bivariate Relationships

Throughout this text, we have stressed how important a visual check of statistical findings can be. Correlations are no exception, and a visual check of relationships can be helpful in understanding the existence and nature of the relationship. A good visual display of the correlational relationship is a scatterplot. This is simply a two-dimensional plot between two or more variables of interest, indicating how the data are spread between the variables. When the interaction between two variables is being considered, it is known as a bivariate relationship (*bi* meaning two). **Figure 9-1** is an example scatterplot showing the relationship between age and depression.

When a scatterplot shows a pattern where the data points are moving in the same direction (i.e., one variable increases as the other increases), as in Figure 9-1, we say that the variables are positively related. However, we say that the variables are negatively related if the data points move in the opposite direction (i.e., one variable increases as the other decreases) as in **Figure 9-2**. If the variables are not related, the data points are scattered all over the place with no pattern (**Figure 9-3**).

Figure 9-1

Example scatterplot between age and depression showing a positive relationship.

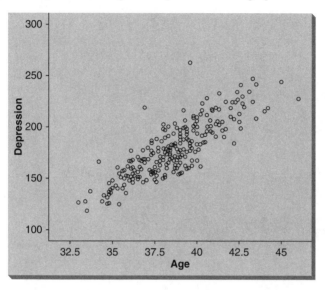

Figure 9-2

Example scatterplot showing a negative relationship.

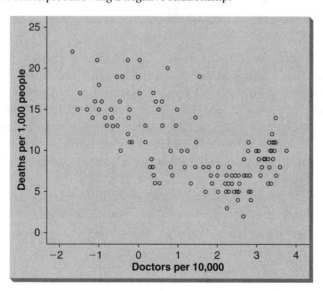

Figure 9-3

Example scatterplot showing no relationship.

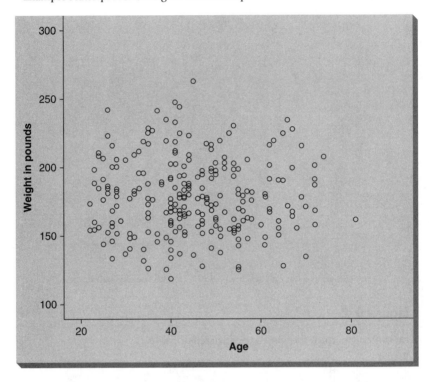

Scatterplots allow us to look at the relationships between variables with visual ease, but a visual inspection can also be somewhat subjective when the relationship is not strongly positive, not strongly negative, or not related. In addition, it will be difficult to precisely describe the relationship and the strength of the relationship shown in the scatterplot. We need some kind of numeric measurement to define both the direction and strength of the relationship to better understand the nature of it.

The simplest way to look at the relationship between variables is to determine whether the two variables covary. The measurement is called **covariance** and can be found using the following formula:

$$\text{Covariance} = \frac{\Sigma (x - \bar{x})(y - \bar{y})}{N - 1}$$

To explain how covariance is computed, let us consider the following data set:

- Number of years in employment (x): 5 2 4 3 1
- Level of job satisfaction (y): 6 9 4 7 2

x	y	$x - \bar{x}$	$y - \bar{y}$	$(x - \bar{x})(y - \bar{y})$	
5	6	2	0.4	0.8	Covariance =
2	9	−1	3.4	−3.4	$\sqrt{\dfrac{3}{4}} = 0.75$
4	4	1	−1.6	−1.6	
3	7	0	1.4	0	
1	2	−2	−3.6	7.2	
$\bar{x} = 3$	$\bar{y} = 5.6$			$\sum (x - \bar{x})(y - \bar{y}) = 3$	

First, you need to calculate means of both variables, x and y, for each subject. You will then subtract the corresponding mean from each and every data value to calculate deviations between a data value and the mean for both variables. Finally, dividing a product between deviations in x and deviations in y with one less of sample size should produce a covariance.

Covariance for the above data set turned out to be 0.75, but what does this mean? Covariance can range from negative infinity to positive infinity and tells us how the two variables of interest are related to each other. Whether a covariance is positive or negative tells us whether the relationship is positive or negative. When a covariance is zero, it means that the two variables are not related. Therefore, our example covariance of 0.75 indicates that our variables, the number of years in employment and level of job satisfaction, are positively related, yet the relationship is very weak as the covariance measure is very close to zero.

The interpretation of covariance seems relatively easy, but there is a major drawback of using covariance as a measure of relationship. Covariance allows us to look at how the variables are related, but it is not a standardized measure. In other words, the measure depends on the measurement scale, and it may not allow for comparisons between one covariance and another. Therefore, we need a standardized measure of relationship to allow us to make such a comparison, and **correlation** is such a measure.

Pearson Correlation Coefficient

Correlation is a standardized measure of the relationship between two or more variables and can be found using the following formula:

$$\text{Correlation} = \frac{\sum (x - \bar{x})(y - \bar{y})}{(N - 1)S_x S_y}$$

where S_x is the standard deviation of x and S_y is the standard deviation of y. When we are dealing with a population, correlation is denoted as ρ, but it is denoted as r when we are dealing with a sample. More precisely, the coefficient in the above equation is known as the Pearson correlation coefficient.

As the correlation becomes a standardized measure of the relationship, it can make scale-free comparison between coefficients and ranges between -1 and $+1$. A coefficient of -1 indicates a perfect negative relationship, meaning that a variable goes down with exactly the same unit change as the other variable goes up, while a coefficient of $+1$ indicates a perfect positive relationship, meaning that a variable goes up as well with exactly the same unit change as the other variable goes up. A coefficient of 0 indicates no relationship between the two variables.

When interpreting a correlation coefficient, a general rule, as shown in **Figure 9-4**, can be applied. However, significance of the correlation coefficient should always be interpreted along with the corresponding value of the correlation coefficient, since the interpretation can be sample specific. SPSS will perform a t-test on a correlation coefficient to see if it is significant for a given sample.

Figure 9-4

Interpreting a correlation coefficient.

Correlation:
−0 and 0.1: no relationship
−0.1 and 0.3: low relationship
−0.3 and 0.5: medium relationship
−0.5 and 0.8: high relationship
>−0.8: very high relationship

Figure 9-5

Selecting correlation in SPSS.

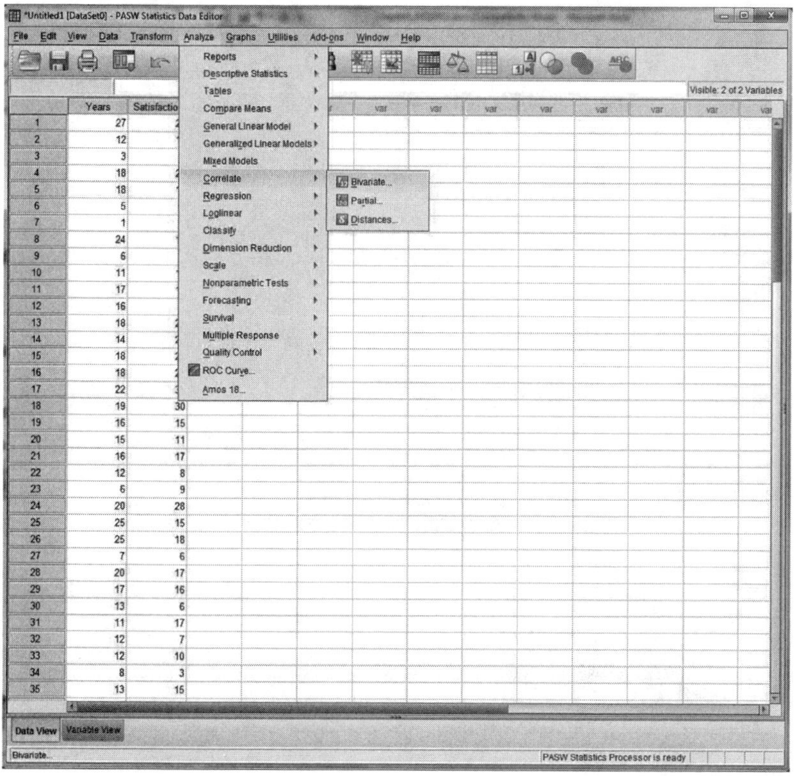

To use the Pearson correlation coefficient in SPSS, you will go to Analyze > Correlates > Bivariates as shown in **Figure** 9-5. In the Bivariate Correlations dialogue box, you will select the variables you are interested in investigating a relationship between and move them over to the right window by clicking the arrow button in the middle as shown in **Figure** 9-6. Pearson's coefficient is checked by default in this dialogue box, so you should leave it if you are not violating parametric assumptions. Clicking "OK" will then produce the output of requested correlation coefficients. Example output is shown in **Table** 9-1.

The Pearson correlation coefficient between the number of years in the current job and the level of satisfaction is .694; this indicates that

Figure 9-6

Defining the variables to compute correlation coefficients in SPSS.

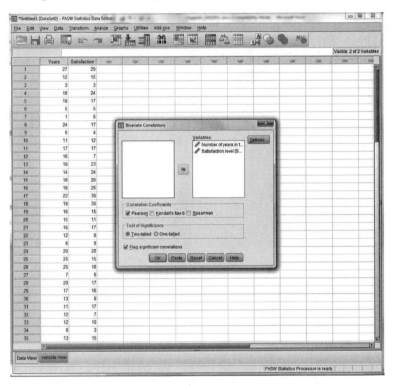

there is a positive relationship between the two variables: the level of satisfaction goes up as the number of years in the current job increases. Note that the corresponding significance *p*-value of .000 in the table indicates that this relationship is statistically significant.

There are two important things to note when interpreting correlation coefficient. The first is that we cannot conclude causality from correlation coefficient. Correlation coefficients only tell us whether or not the two variables are related; it does not imply **causality** (i.e., change on one variable causes the other variable to change). For example, having a correlation coefficient of .75 between weight and systolic blood pressure implies that the two variables are positively related, but it does not say anything about heavier weight causing increased systolic blood pressure. We should keep this in mind, as confusing correlation with causality is one of the commonly made mistakes.

Table	
9-1	**Example Output for Pearson Correlation Coefficient**

Correlations

		Number of Years in the Current Job	Satisfaction Level
Number of years in the current job	Pearson correlation	1	.694**
	Sig. (2-tailed)		.000
	N	89	89
Satisfaction level	Pearson correlation	.694**	1
	Sig. (2-tailed)	.000	
	N	89	89

** Correlation is significant at the 0.01 level (2-tailed).

The second important thing to note about the correlation coefficient is that the ratio of differences between and/or among correlation coefficients cannot be expressed. For example, a correlation coefficient of .50 does not means the relationship is twice as strong as a correlation coefficient of .25.

Coefficient of Determination

A correlation coefficient can be squared to provide additional information. A squared correlation coefficient is called a **coefficient of determination** and tells us how much variability in one variable is explained or shared by the other variable. For example, let us suppose that we are interested in looking at the relationship between the number of nursing staff at a nursing home and the quality of nursing care. Let us suppose that we found a correlation coefficient between the two of .39. Taking a square of this correlation coefficient, we get $(.39)^2 = 0.1521$; this means that 15.21% of the variability in quality of nursing care is explained by the number of staff at a nursing home. Perhaps more importantly, this also means that the remaining 84.79% of variability in quality of care is contributed by something other than the number of staff. The coefficient of determination can be useful in determining how important the relationship between the variables is; the larger the coefficient, the more the variables explain each other.

Spearman's Rho and Kendall's Tau

Pearson's correlation coefficient is a parametric correlation coefficient, which means that it requires parametric assumptions such as the normality assumption. When parametric assumptions are not met (such as nonnormally distributed variables or ordinal variables), the Pearson correlation coefficient cannot be used to examine the relationship between the variables. Two alternatives to Pearson's correlation coefficient in this situation are Spearman's rho and Kendall's tau. Both coefficients are calculated by first ranking the data and then applying the same equation we used for Pearson's correlation coefficient. We will not discuss the detailed computation of these two statistics, but the interpretation of coefficients is done in the same manner as before.

To request either Spearman's rho or Kendall's tau in SPSS, you will go to Analyze > Correlates > Bivariates as shown in **Figure 9-7**. In the Bivariate Correlations dialogue box, you will select the variables that you are interested in investigating the relationship between and move them over to the right window by clicking the arrow button in the middle as shown in **Figure 9-8**. Pearson is checked by default in this box, but you should uncheck it and select Spearman and Kendall's tau-b instead if you are violating required parametric assumptions. Clicking "OK" will then produce the output of requested correlation coefficients. An example output is shown in **Table 9-2**.

Figure 9-7

Selecting Spearman's and Kendall's correlation coefficients in SPSS.

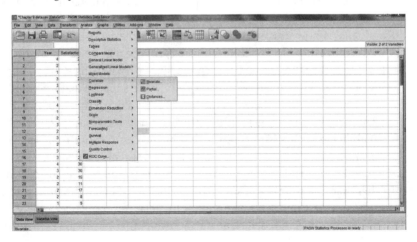

Figure 9-8

Defining variables for Spearman's and Kendall's correlation coefficients in SPSS.

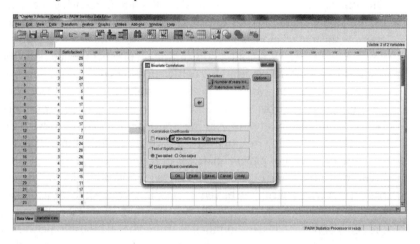

Table			Satisfaction Level	Year
9-2	**Example Output for Spearman's and Kendall's Correlation Coefficients**			
Correlations				
			Satisfaction Level	**Year**
Kendall's tau_b	Satisfaction level	Correlation coefficient	1.000	.392[**]
		Sig. (2-tailed)		.000
		N	89	89
	Year	Correlation coefficient	.392[**]	1.000
		Sig. (2-tailed)	.000	
		N	89	89
Spearman's rho	Satisfaction level	Correlation coefficient	1.000	.509[**]
		Sig. (2-tailed)		.000
		N	89	89
	Year	Correlation coefficient	.509[**]	1.000
		Sig. (2-tailed)	.000	
		N	89	89

[**] Correlation is significant at the 0.01 level (2-tailed).

Partial Correlation

Oftentimes, there may be other variables that are influencing the main relationship you are currently investigating. If this is the case, you cannot examine the true relationship between the two variables of interests unless you do something with regard to the unwanted or other variable(s) in the relationship. A **partial correlation coefficient** allows us to look at the true relationship between two variables after controlling for the influence of a third/unwanted variable (i.e., the effect of that variable is held constant). Let us assume that a nurse practitioner (NP) is interested in studying the relationship between a treatment and a patient outcome, but the NP believes that the level of patient anxiety is also influencing the relationship between treatment and outcome. If the NP does not control for the effect of patient anxiety, the result can be very misleading because it will not account for the true relationship between the two variables. The NP should control the effect of patient anxiety and then examine the relationship between a treatment and the patient outcome. Partial correlation allows us to do this.

To explain partial correlation a bit more, let us consider **Figure** 9-9. The first diagram shows the relationship between patient outcome and

Figure 9-9

Example diagram of partial correlation.

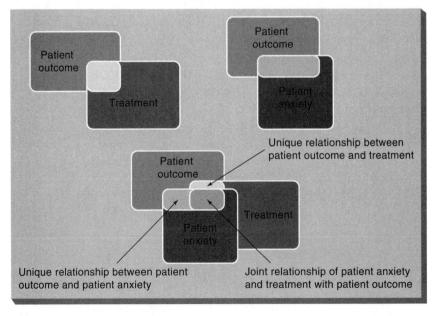

treatment, and the second diagram shows the relationship between patient outcome and patient anxiety. When we combine those two diagrams together, you will notice that the double shaded area in the middle is the portion of variability in patient outcome that is shared by both patient anxiety and a treatment. Therefore, there is not a unique relationship between a treatment and patient outcome, and patient anxiety should be removed from the rectangle of the first diagram. What is left will be the true relationship between a treatment and patient outcome.

To obtain a partial correlation coefficient in SPSS, go to Analyze > Correlate > Partial as shown in **Figure 9-10**. In the Partial Correlations dialogue box, you will select the variables you are interested in investigating a relationship between and move them over to the upper

Figure 9-10

Selecting partial correlation in SPSS.

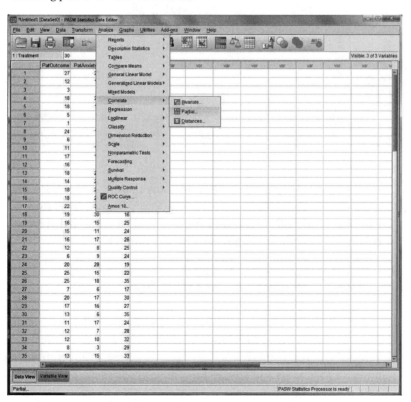

Figure 9-11

Defining the variables to compute partial correlation coefficient in SPSS.

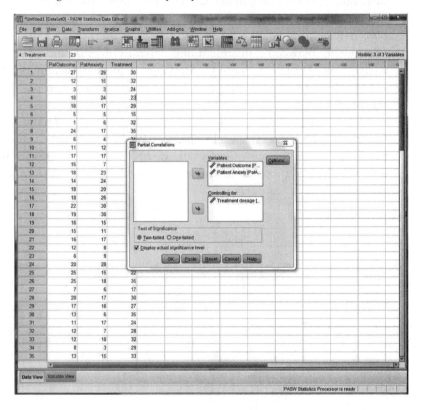

window by clicking the arrow button in the middle. You will also move a variable to control to the lower window as shown in **Figure 9-11**. Clicking "OK" will then produce the output of requested correlation coefficients. Example output is shown in **Table 9-3**.

Correlation Coefficient as an Effect Size

Correlation coefficient is actually one of the commonly used measures of effect size. When a correlation coefficient is used as an effect size, a value of ±.1 represents a small effect, ±.3 represents a medium effect, and ±.5 represents a large effect.

Table					
9-3	**Example Output for Partial Correlation Coefficient**				

Correlations				
Control Variables			**Patient Outcome**	**Patient Anxiety**
Treatment dosage	Patient outcome	Correlation	1.000	.694
		Significance (2-tailed)		.000
		df	0	86
	Patient anxiety	Correlation	.694	1.000
		Significance (2-tailed)	.000	
		df	86	0

Reporting Correlation Coefficients

You should include the size of the relationship between variables and its associated significance when reporting the results of correlation coefficients if you are to report the results in American Psychological Association (APA) format. Some important things to remember when reporting correlation coefficients are: (a) you should not include zero in front of the decimal, (b) all correlation coefficients should be reported in two decimals, and (c) the significance of correlation coefficients should be indicated using a different number of asterisks if you decide to report them in a table format. Two examples of reporting correlation coefficients are shown below.

1. There was a significant negative relationship between surgery outcome and anxiety, $r = -.38, p < .001$.

2.

	Anxiety	**Surgery Outcome**
Anxiety	1	$-.38^{***}$
Surgery outcome	$-.38^{***}$	1
Note: *** $p < .001$		

SUMMARY

Examining relationships between variables is one of the most common approaches in hypothesis testing. Looking at relationships through a visual display like a scatterplot is a simple way of examining the relationship between variables. However, it can be somewhat subjective to determine whether variables are related to each other solely based on a visual display.

Covariance is a measure that allows us to look at relationships between variables, but it is not a standardized measure that allows comparisons across the data measured on different types of scales. Correlation allows us to overcome this pitfall and to look at relationship in a standard and more precise way.

We can use bivariate correlation coefficients if the researcher is interested in whether the two variables are related to each other. We can also use the partial correlation coefficient if there seems to be a third/unwanted variable that may influence the relationship between the variables of interest.

As Pearson correlation coefficients require parametric assumptions such as normality, either Spearman's rho or Kendall's tau correlation coefficients should be used if there are violations of assumptions.

The correlation coefficient is also a type of the commonly reported effect size and a value of $\pm.1$ represents a small effect, $\pm.3$ represents a medium effect, and $\pm.5$ represents a large effect.

When reporting correlation coefficients, the size of the relationship between variables and its associated significance should also be included.

Critical Thinking Questions www

1. It is not correct to say that a correlation coefficient of .60 is twice as strong as a coefficient of .30. Explain why.
2. Covariance is a measure of relationships, but it is treated as a crude measure of relationships when compared to correlation. Explain why.
3. Write a research question or hypothesis that could be answered/tested using a correlation coefficient.
4. Under what circumstances should we use Spearman's coefficient? Pearson's coefficient?

5. Use the data file called *SBP.sav* (found on the Student Companion Website using the access code card from the front of this text) to create a scatterplot, compute a correlation coefficient, and determine if there is a relationship between age and SBP (systolic blood pressure). Report the results in APA format.
6. In the following case study, identify the independent and dependent variables and the type of correlation coefficient used. What conclusion may be made about the direction and strength of the associations identified?

Drs. Manojlovich, Antonakos, and Ronis (2009) published the following study in the *American Journal of Critical Care*. In the study, they studied the association between nurse and physician communication and patient outcomes.

Case Study

Manojlovich, M., Antonakos, C. L., & Ronis, D. L (2009). Intensive care units, communication between nurses and physicians, and patient's outcomes. *American Journal of Critical Care, 18*(1), 21–30.

Objectives: To determine the relationships between patients' outcomes and (1) nurses' perceptions of elements of communication between nurses and physicians and (2) characteristics of the practice environment.

Methods: A cross-sectional survey design was used. Information on ventilator-associated pneumonia, bloodstream infection associated with a central catheter, and pressure ulcers was collected from 25 intensive care units in southeastern Michigan. Simultaneously, 462 nurses in those units (response rate, 53.3%) were anonymously surveyed. The Conditions for Work Effectiveness Questionnaire-II and the Practice Environment Scale of the Nursing Work Index were used to measure characteristics of the practice environment. The Intensive Care Unit Nurse–Physician Questionnaire was used to measure communication between nurses and physicians. Statistical tests included correlation and multiple regression. Analyses were conducted at the unit level.

Results: Unit response rates varied from 6% to 100%. Together, variability in understanding communication and capacity utilization were predictive of 27% of the variance in ventilator-associated pneumonia. Timeliness of communication was inversely related to pressure ulcers ($r = -0.38$; $P = .06$).

Conclusions: Not all elements of communication were related to the selected adverse outcomes. The connection between characteristics of the practice environment at the unit level and adverse outcomes remains elusive.

Self-Quiz www

1. Which of the following correlation coefficients represents the strongest relationship?
   a. $+.14$
   b. $+.82$
   c. $-.02$
   d. $-.34$
   e. $+.56$
2. True or false: If a correlation coefficient is -1.00, it means that the two variables will move in opposite directions with an equal unit change.
3. True or false: The correlation coefficient between age and depression is $+.85$. Since this coefficient is high enough, one can conclude that aging will cause increasing depression.

REFERENCES

Burtson, P. L., & Stichler, J. F. (2010). Nursing work environment and nurse caring: Relationship among motivational factors. *Journal of Advanced Nursing, 66*(8), 1819–1831. doi: 0.1111/j.1365-2648.2010.05336.x

Manojlovich, M., Antonakos, C. L., & Ronis, D. L. (2009). Intensive care units, communication between nurses and physicians, and patient's outcomes. *American Journal of Critical Care, 18*(1), 21–30.

Mor, V., Intrator, O., Feng, Z., & Grabowski, D. C. (2010). The revolving door of rehospitalization from skilled nursing facilities. *Health Affairs, 29*(1), 57–64.

Chapter

10 | Modeling Relationships

Learning Objectives

The principal goal of this chapter is to explain how the relationships between variables can be taken one step further to predict and estimate the variation on the dependent variable when information is known for the independent variable(s). This chapter will prepare you to:

- Explain the concepts of simple and multiple linear regression and logistic regression
- Compute the necessary regression values to analyze the data and make predictions
- Evaluate the assumptions in regression analysis
- Choose the right regression analysis for a given research problem/question
- Make inferences based on a regression model and regression coefficients
- Interpret coefficient of determination
- Formulate a regression model and make predictions
- Understand the different types of models and the selection procedures
- Correctly report the regression findings in APA style
- Understand how predictions apply in nursing practice

Key Terms www

Enter method

Goodness of fit

Hierarchical method

Linearity

Logistic regression

Method of least squares

Multicollinearity

Percentage of variance

Predictor variable

R-square

Regression model

Residual

Stepwise method

INTRODUCTION

We have learned that correlations tell us whether variables of interest are related or associated with one another, and if so, how strong the relationship is. For example, a correlation coefficient of $+.50$ tells us that the variables are positively and moderately related to each other. Correlations and their strength provide important information about clinical phenomena that we are just beginning to explore. In correlation, we do not specify which are the independent and dependent variables, and all we are interested in is whether or not the variables are related. However, understanding how variables are related is usually a precursor to a more important level of understanding: prediction of the dependent variable by one or more independent variables.

Let us consider a study examining the relationship between fat and protein in the human body, and the correlation coefficient indicated that fat and protein are negatively related (i.e., protein level will increase as fat content decreases in the human body). Depending upon how strong the relationship is, we could then try to estimate or predict the value of one variable using the value of the other variable; in this case, does the level of protein predict the level of fat in body composition? Obviously, the estimation or prediction will be more accurate when the relationship is stronger. This is what regression analysis does!

In clinical practice and research it is often not enough to understand that a relationship exists between variables. We often need to know how much influence is exerted by the independent variable on the dependent variable—in other words, we want to know what proportion or **percentage of variance** on the dependent variable is contributed by any one independent variable. For example, we might ask, "How much variance in the proportion of body fat is predicted by body mass index?" The purpose of such research is to outline initial thinking about how to regulate phenomena. Similarly, in evidence-based practice, we are often interested in predictions so that we can change practices that influence patient outcomes. To take an example in evidence-based practice, we might ask, "How much variance in hospital-acquired urinary tract infections is attributable to the length of time that urinary catheters are in place?"

Case Study

Aggar, C., Ronaldson, S., & Cameron, I. D. (2010). Reactions to caregiving of frail, older persons predict depression. *International Journal of Mental Health Nursing, 19,* 409–415.

In 2010, researchers Christina Aggar, Susan Ronaldson, and Ian D. Cameron published a study that examined whether or not depression could be predicted from caregivers' responses to caregiving for frail elders living in a community setting. They hypothesized that five dimensions—impact on the carer's usual activities, financial strain, energy and physical capacity to provide care, perceived family support, and self-esteem—would predict depression and anxiety in caregivers. They designed a cross-sectional predictive study with 93 caregivers and used multiple linear regression analysis to test the null hypothesis. They found that impact on usual activities and energy/physical capacity predicted 46% of the variance on depression and 42% of the variance on anxiety. Aggar, Ronaldson, and Cameron (2010) conclude that future research and interventions should focus on supporting caregivers' needs around daily activities and health. This study is an excellent example of how prediction of dependent variables using linear regression analysis helps both researchers and clinicians make informed decisions about logical next steps.

DOING AND INTERPRETING SIMPLE LINEAR REGRESSION

To explain how regression analysis is performed and to understand the underlying principles, let us recall our college algebra course. Specifically, let us turn our attention to the **linear** equation modeling that we used to characterize the relationship between x and y. We can understand that relationship as the best fit using the following equation:

$$Y = a + b \times X$$

where a is the y-intercept of a line and b is the slope of the line.

In regression analysis, we are doing exactly the same thing: trying to fit a line that best describes the data. However, we introduce an error term in the above equation since we are predicting/estimating the value of a dependent variable using information from an independent variable (because no estimation or prediction will be perfect!). Then, the linear line equation becomes:

$$Y = (a + b \times X) + error$$

In this equation, $a + b \times X$ is called the model, and we use it to predict the value of the dependent variable based on knowns about the independent variable. Error is the difference between the actual value and our estimate. When the model is able to explain the data and minimize error, the estimation or prediction will be accurate, but the opposite is also correct—large errors or inability to explain most of the data limits what we can say about predictions.

In prediction, regression analysis uses the **method of least squares**. In this approach, the idea is to find the line that best fits the data with the least amount of vertical distance between the fitted line and the actual data among many lines that could be fitted to the data, or **residual**. To explain residual further, let us consider **Figure 10-1**. The vertical lines between each data point and the fitted line through the data points represent residuals, and the least squares method is designed to find a line that minimizes the sum of these residuals for each and every data point. The better fit of the line through the data and the smaller the sum of residuals, the better predictive value of the model. In other words, the better the line fits, the more accurately it tells about

Figure 10-1

Method of least squares in graph.

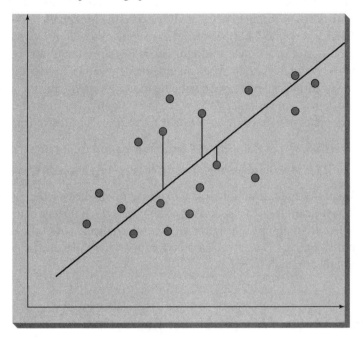

how much variance the independent variable explains or predicts on the dependent variable.

Overall Model Fit

Once the line has been fitted to the data, one way to examine how good the fitted line is for estimation or prediction is to evaluate the goodness of fit. Regression analysis will calculate what is called R^2, or **R-square**, simply a square of a correlation coefficient, and we can use this statistic to evaluate goodness of fit. **Goodness of fit** is the ratio of the percentage of variability explained by the fitted model (line) over the total variability in the data. The more variability in the data that can be explained by the line and the more accurate our model is, the higher this R^2 statistic gets. For example, a model with R-square of 75% will have better fit than a model with R^2 of 42% since the former explains more variability and minimizes the amount of variability we cannot explain (i.e., error).

Parameters

Along with goodness of fit of the model, we also need to examine the statistical significance of the predictor (i.e., the independent variable). There is a relationship between the overall goodness of it and the significance of individual **predictor variables**, since the model will contain good predictability when an independent variable is significant for predication (i.e., it is a good variable to use for predicting the value of the dependent variable). SPSS will test the significance of an individual independent variable using t-test; the hypotheses for this t-test are:

H_0: $\beta = 0$ or independent variable is not useful for prediction

H_a: $\beta \neq 0$ or independent variable is useful for prediction

The independent variable is said to be a good predictor when the result is significant (i.e., the associated p-value with the independent variable is less than alpha) and not such a good predictor when the result is not significant (i.e., associated p-value with the independent variable is larger than alpha).

General Steps of Simple Linear Regression

In general, the steps for conducting a simple linear regression are as follows. First, you will draw and examine a scatterplot of the data and visually check the strength of the linear relationship between variables. Second, you will compute the correlation coefficients as a numerical verification of what you saw in the scatterplot if the relationship in the plot appears relatively strong. Finally, if the correlation coefficient is significant, you will try to fit the best line of prediction through regression analysis.

To help explain simple linear regression, let us think about the following example and see how a regression analysis is done in SPSS. A nurse researcher is interested in examining the relationship between gross domestic product (GDP) per capita and life expectancy in a number of countries, and in predicting life expectancy with GDP per capita if they seem to be related. The data for this example are shown in **Figure 10-2**, and a scatterplot between GDP per capita and life expectancy is shown in **Figure 10-3**.

Figure 10-2

Screen shot of the data.

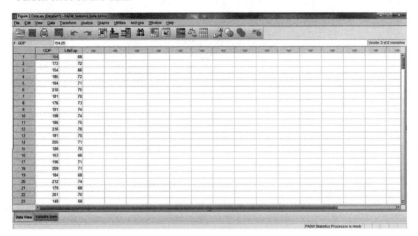

Figure 10-3

Scatterplot between GDP per capita and life expectancy.

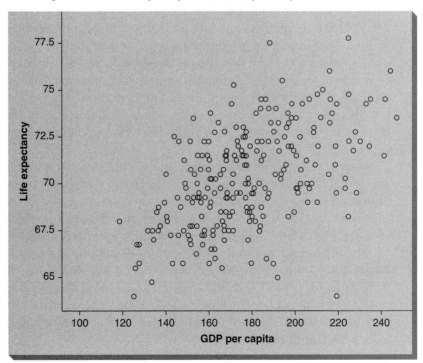

Table			
10-1	**Correlation Coefficient Between GDP per Capita and Life Expectancy**		
Correlations			
		GDP per Capita	**Life Expectancy**
GDP per capita	Pearson correlation	1	.535[**]
	Sig. (2-tailed)		.000
	N	246	246
Life expectancy	Pearson correlation	.535[**]	1
	Sig. (2-tailed)	.000	
	N	246	246
[**] Correlation is significant at the 0.01 level (2-tailed).			

The scatterplot shows a somewhat moderate positive relationship, where life expectancy increases as GDP per capita increases, so let us proceed to computing the correlation coefficient to see if the relationship is significant enough for prediction. The SPSS output for the correlation coefficient for these data is shown in **Table 10-1**. From the table we can see that the relationship between GDP per capita and life expectancy is statistically significant and moderately strong, $r = .54$, $p < .001$. Therefore, we have a good reason to try fitting a simple regression line and determine if we may predict life expectancy with per capita GDP.

To conduct simple linear regression analysis in SPSS, you will go to Analyze > Regression > Linear as shown in **Figure 10-4**. In the Linear Regression dialogue box, you will select the variables you are interested in fitting a prediction line between and move an independent variable into "Independent(s)" and a dependent variable into "Dependent" by clicking the corresponding arrow buttons in the middle, as shown in **Figure 10-5**. For methods, "Enter" is selected by default and we will leave it as is for now. (The methods will be explained further in a later section for multiple linear regression.) Clicking "OK" will then produce the output of requested regression analysis. The example output is shown in **Table 10-2**.

Figure 10-4

Selecting regression in SPSS.

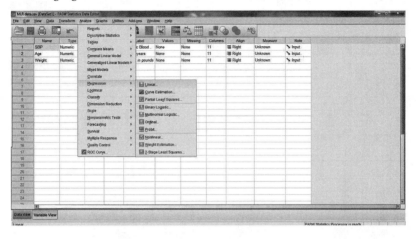

The first section in Table 10-2 is for overall fit of the model; you can see that the correlation coefficient between GDP per capita and life expectancy is .535, as previously calculated. In the same section, we see the value of R^2 is .287, which tells us that GDP per capita explains about 28.7% of the variability in life expectancy, and there is 71.3% of the variability in life expectancy that cannot be explained by GDP per capita by itself.

Figure 10-5

Defining variables for regression analysis in SPSS.

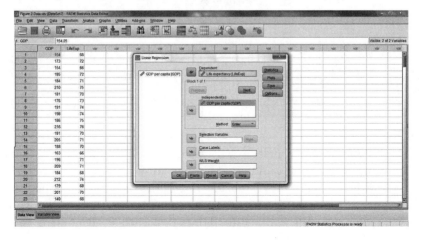

Table	
10-2	Example Regression Analysis Output

Model Summary

Model	R	R-Square	Adjusted R-Square	Std. Error of the Estimate
1	.535[a]	.287	.284	2.220

[a] Predictors: (Constant), GDP per capita

ANOVA[b]

Model		Sum of Squares	df	Mean Square	F	Sig.
1	Regression	483.451	1	483.451	98.068	.000[a]
	Residual	1202.857	244	4.930		
	Total	1686.308	245			

[a] Predictors: (Constant), GDP per capita
[b] Dependent variable: Life expectancy

Coefficients[a]

Model		Unstandardized Coefficients		Standardized Coefficients		
		B	Std. Error	Beta	t	Sig.
1	(Constant)	60.840	.968		62.851	.000
	GDP per capita	.053	.005	.535	9.903	.000

[a] Dependent variable: Life expectancy

You may ask yourself now, "What is a good value for R^2?" Is the value of .287 we found good enough for a prediction model? The answer is, "It depends!" In some disciplines or in investigating some phenomena, an R^2 of 75% may not be high enough to make a good prediction, while in other disciplines or particular phenomena an R^2

of 25% may be high enough. Evaluating R-square may also depend on the literature; for example, R^2 of 25% can be important and significant enough if others doing the same type of research have reported 5–10% R^2 in the past. However, R^2 of 75% may not be important and significant enough if others doing the same type of research have consistently reported R^2 of 85% or above. It may also depend on the sample or population under study or whether or not any research has been done on these variables before. Rejecting the null hypothesis in regression analysis is a matter of the strength of the R-square and significance of the independent variable situated in the larger context of the research or evidence already available.

The next section in Table 10-2 is an analysis of variance (ANOVA) presenting the various sums of squares (i.e., variability) as well as degrees of freedom. Sums of squares for regression are the amount of variability that is explained by the current model, and sums of squares for residual is the amount of variability that is not explained by the current model. When you combine the two, you should get the total sums of squares. The degree of freedom for regression is 1, since we are fitting only one regression line, and the total degrees of freedom is equal to the sample size minus 1. Then, the degrees of freedom for residual will be the total degrees of freedom minus 1, which is equal to 244 in this example. Mean squares can be found by dividing sums of squares by corresponding degrees of freedom, and F-ratio is found by the ratio between mean squares for regression and that for residual. This F-ratio and associated p-value indicate that this model is a good prediction model with a significant p-value under the hypotheses of

H_0: this model is not a good prediction model

H_a: this model is a good and significant prediction model

The last section shown in Table 10-2 is the results of significance testing of the independent variable in predicting a dependent variable. The ANOVA section of Table 10-2 tells us whether or not a prediction model fitted is a good model, but it is not necessarily reporting whether or not an independent variable is a good predictor variable of the dependent variable. As stated before, SPSS will perform a t-test for an independent variable, and an independent variable is said to be a good predictor if p-value of this table is less than alpha. For our example, associated *p*-value is less than alpha; therefore GDP per capita is determined to be a good predictor variable of life expectancy.

The values in Table 10-2 can be used to create a prediction line for the data. By plugging unstandardized coefficients (B) into a regression equation, $y = a + b \times x$, we obtain

$$Life\ expectancy = 60.84 + 0.053 \times GDP\ per\ capita$$

This equation then can be used to predict life expectancy if we know the value of GDP per capita. For example, the value of life expectancy of a country with GDP per capita of 199 will be

$$Life\ expectancy = 60.84 + 0.053 \times GDP\ per\ capita$$
$$= 60.84 + 0.053 \times 199$$
$$\approx 71.57$$

Reporting Simple Linear Regression

Reporting regression analysis results can be done simply in a table format that includes, at minimum, the unstandardized coefficients (B), standard error of unstandardized coefficients (B), standardized coefficients (β), and some overall statistics about the fitted model, such as R^2. Reporting for our example is shown in **Table 10-3**. Results indicate that GDP per capita is a significant predictor of life expectancy with GDP per capita sharing 29% of the variability in life expectancy.

Table			
10-3	**Example Reporting of Simple Linear Regression Results**		
	B	*SE (B)*	*β*
Constant	60.84	.97	
GDP per capita	.05	.01	.54*
*Note: R^2 = .29; * p < .001*			

MULTIPLE LINEAR REGRESSION

Introduction

Multiple linear regression is basically an extension of simple linear regression, where two or more independent variables, either continuous or categorical, are jointly used to predict a single dependent variable. An example from the case study discussed earlier may help illustrate this concept. Aggar et al. (2010) examined the predictive capacity of five independent variables: (1) financial strain, (2) energy, (3) physical capacity to provide care, (4) perceived family support, and (5) self-esteem on a single dependent variable, either depression or anxiety. Recall the equation for simple linear regression:

$$y = a + bx + \varepsilon$$

Now that we have more than one variable to use for prediction, this equation is extended to

$$y = b_0 + b_1 x_1 + b_2 x_2 + \cdots + b_n x_n + \varepsilon$$

where y is the dependent variable, b_0 is the y-intercept, b_1 is the *partial* regression coefficient of the first independent variable (x_1), b_2 is the *partial* regression coefficient of the second independent variable (x_2), b_n is the *partial* regression coefficient of the nth independent variable (x_n), and ε_1 is the error. Note here that we call b_1 *partial* regression coefficient because it is not a solely unique contribution of corresponding independent variables. Rather, it is the additional amount of contribution by an independent variable after the other independent variables went into the model and explained variability within the dependent variable. With this model, our goal is to find the best linear combination of independent variables that jointly predict a dependent variable. However, we are fitting a plane on a three- or more dimensional space rather than a linear line on a two-dimensional space since we have more than one independent variable to use for prediction. A visual explanation of the difference between simple linear regression and multiple linear regression is shown in **Figure 10-6**.

In simple linear regression analysis, we were interested in the ability of a single independent variable to predict a single dependent variable. In human research and evidence-based practice, however, it is rare that

Figure 10-6

Difference between simple linear regression and multiple linear regression.

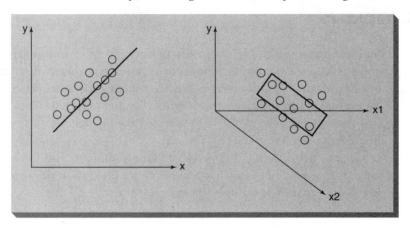

phenomena are composed of only one independent variable and one dependent variable. In most cases we know that multiple variables are involved. Multiple linear regression becomes useful in examining the ability of two or more independent variables to predict one dependent variable.

Doing and Interpreting Multiple Linear Regression

To explain multiple linear regressions, let us consider the following example data set, taken from Cengage Learning (2010; http://college. cengage.com/mathematics/brase/understandable_statistics/7e/students/ datasets/mlr/frames/frame.html). Click on "Systolic Blood Pressure Data" in the list in the center of the page to show the data file download options on the right. There are three variables: systolic blood pressure, age in years, and weight in pounds. Our goal is to find the best linear combination of age in years and weight in pounds to predict systolic blood pressure.

As always, the first step is to check whether the required assumptions are met; the following assumptions should be met for multiple linear regressions:

- **Linearity:** The relationship between the dependent variable and independent variables should be linear. As the title says, we are trying to fit a linear relationship, not a nonlinear one. As usual, this assumption can be checked with a scatterplot.

- **Independence:** The values of dependent variables are assumed to be independent, meaning that none of the values are from the same person. This assumption can be checked with Durbin–Watson statistics and can be requested as an option in the regression window. If the value of that statistic is around +2, the assumption is said to be met. Otherwise, you will be violating the assumption. **Table 10-4** shows the critical values of this statistic and can be used as a guideline to determine the violation of this assumption. If the statistic is outside of the interval, you violate this assumption.

- **Normality:** All variables should follow multivariate normal distribution. Multivariate normal assumption is tricky to check, but can be investigated with a histogram, skewness and kurtosis, a P-P plot, or statistical tests such as the Kolmogorov–Smirnov test or Shapiro–Wilk test. These tests hypothesize that the variable is normally distributed for a null hypothesis and that the variable is not normally distributed for an alternative hypothesis. When the result is significant (i.e., *p*-value is less than alpha), it means that the variable is not normally distributed. Otherwise, the variable is normally distributed.

- **Equal variance:** The variance of error should be equal at each level of independent variables, and this assumption can be checked with a residual plot, which also can be requested as an option in the regression window. You should not see data values scattered without any specific pattern if you were to meet this assumption. If you see a specific pattern—like a megaphone effect, where the range of the data values increases depending upon the location—you are violating this assumption.

- **No multicollinearity:** Independent variables should not be highly correlated with each other, and if they are highly correlated (over .85) they may be measuring the same value. The final goal of multiple linear regressions is to find the best model of prediction with the lowest possible number of variables and maximum explanation about the data. We should examine for multicollinearity and remove one of the variables if it is present.

Table											
10-4	**Critical Values for Durbin–Watson Statistic**										

Sample Size	Probability in Lower Tail (Significance Level = α)	k = Number of Regressors (Excluding the Intercept)									
		1		2		3		4		5	
		d_L	d_U	d_L	d_U	d_L	d_U	d_L	d_U	d_L	d_U
15	.01	.81	1.07	.70	1.25	.59	1.46	.49	1.70	.39	1.96
	.025	.95	1.23	.83	1.40	.71	1.61	.59	1.84	.48	2.09
	.05	1.08	1.36	.95	1.54	.82	1.75	.69	1.97	.56	2.21
20	.01	.95	1.15	.86	1.27	.77	1.41	.63	1.57	.60	1.74
	.025	1.08	1.28	.99	1.41	.89	1.55	.79	1.70	.70	1.87
	.05	1.20	1.41	1.10	1.54	1.00	1.68	.90	1.83	.79	1.99
25	.01	1.05	1.21	.98	1.30	.90	1.41	.83	1.52	.75	1.65
	.025	1.13	1.34	1.10	1.43	1.02	1.54	.94	1.65	.86	1.77
	.05	1.29	1.45	1.21	1.55	1.12	1.66	1.04	1.77	.95	1.89
30	.01	1.13	1.26	1.07	1.34	1.01	1.42	.94	1.51	.88	1.61
	.025	1.25	1.38	1.18	1.46	1.12	1.54	1.05	1.63	.98	1.73
	.05	1.35	1.49	1.28	1.57	1.21	1.65	1.14	1.74	1.07	1.83
40	.01	1.25	1.34	1.20	1.40	1.15	1.46	1.10	1.52	1.05	1.58
	.025	1.35	1.45	1.30	1.51	1.25	1.57	1.20	1.63	1.15	1.69
	.05	1.44	1.54	1.39	1.60	1.34	1.66	1.29	1.72	1.23	1.79
50	.01	1.32	1.40	1.28	1.45	1.24	1.49	1.20	1.54	1.16	1.59
	.025	1.42	1.50	1.38	1.54	1.34	1.59	1.30	1.64	1.26	1.69
	.05	1.50	1.59	1.46	1.63	1.42	1.67	1.38	1.72	1.34	1.77
60	.01	1.38	1.45	1.35	1.48	1.32	1.52	1.28	1.56	1.25	1.60
	.025	1.47	1.54	1.44	1.57	1.40	1.61	1.37	1.65	1.33	1.69
	.05	1.55	1.62	1.51	1.65	1.48	1.69	1.44	1.73	1.41	1.77
80	.01	1.47	1.52	1.44	1.54	1.42	1.57	1.39	1.60	1.36	1.62
	.025	1.54	1.59	1.52	1.62	1.49	1.65	1.47	1.67	1.44	1.70
	.05	1.61	1.66	1.59	1.69	1.56	1.72	1.53	1.74	1.51	1.77
100	.01	1.52	1.56	1.50	1.58	1.48	1.60	1.45	1.63	1.44	1.65
	.025	1.59	1.63	1.57	1.65	1.55	1.67	1.53	1.70	1.51	1.72
	.05	1.65	1.69	1.63	1.72	1.61	1.74	1.59	1.76	1.57	1.78

Source: "Testing for Serial Correlation in Least Squares Regression II" by J. Durbin and G. S. Watson, *Biometrika, Vol.* 38, 1951.

Descriptives

All inferential statistics should begin with descriptive statistics because it provides a feel for the data especially in terms of accuracy. Descriptive statistics can be requested as an option in the regression window, and this should help you understand the results of regression analysis.

Overall Model Fit

Once we find a plane that fits the data, we can examine how good the fitted hyperplane is for estimation or prediction by evaluating the goodness of fit. Regression analysis will output R^2, and we can use this statistic to evaluate goodness of fit. There is no difference in the definition of R-square in multiple linear regression; it is still the ratio of the percentage of variability explained by the fitted model (line) over the total variability in the data. However, this is not the same R^2 as the one we calculated in simple linear regression. Then, it was simply a square of correlation coefficient between the two variables, but R^2 in multiple linear regressions is more than a simple square of correlation coefficient. We have more independent variables to look at, so they should be considered jointly. Due to the complexity of computation, how to calculate R^2 in multiple linear regressions will not be discussed here. However, the interpretation is done in the same manner as before; the higher R^2, the better the model and the greater accuracy of prediction.

The ANOVA table will also be used to check overall fit of the model, and the model is said to be a good one when *F*-ratio comes out to be significant with its associated *p*-value.

Model Parameters

This part of output will tell you whether the independent variables are significant predictors of a dependent variable, and again, there is a relationship between the overall goodness of fit and the significance of each individual predictor variable. The model will contain good predictability when an independent variable is significant for prediction (i.e., it is a good variable to use for predicting the value of dependent variable). SPSS will test the significance of each individual independent variable using a t-test, and hypotheses for these t-tests are:

H_0: $\beta_i = 0$ or independent variable does not predict

H_a: $\beta_i \neq 0$ or independent variable is useful for prediction

The independent variables are said to be good predictors when the result is significant (i.e., the associated p-value with the independent variable is less than alpha) and not such a good predictor when the result is not significant (i.e., the associated p-value with the independent variable is larger than alpha).

Model Selection

Our goal in multiple linear regression is to find the best prediction model with the lowest possible number of independent variables. Having more independent variables as predictors in a model does not mean that it is the best model; it may contain nonsignificant independent variables, which do not do add any predictive strength and therefore are better left out of the model since they will only complicate the model without adding predictive strength. There are three commonly discussed model selection procedures—**enter, hierarchical**, and **stepwise**—and we will cover each one.

Enter Method

This is the default method in regression analysis, and it forces all of the independent variables into the **regression model** at the same time. Then, all parameter estimates are computed and tested for their significance. Since they are forced to enter the model all at once, no modification of the model at the initial step is allowed.

Hierarchical Method

In this method, the researcher can select different blocks of independent variables based on the importance or interest in particular variables. It usually allows us to examine regression parameter estimates in nested data; a common approach is to begin by adding only demographic variables in the first block and then add independent variables of interest to see if these new independent variables add more predictability to what has been explained by demographic variables. As this is a little beyond the scope of this text, we will limit our discussion here.

Stepwise Methods

In these methods, variables are entered into the model based on preset statistical criteria, and there are three different methods of stepwise selection. In **forward selection**, we begin with an empty model with only a constant (i.e., y-intercept). Then, independent variables are added to the model based on their statistical significance, with the most significantly related independent variable entered first, followed by the next most significant and so on. This process continues until the remaining variables are not statistically significant (i.e., associated p-values are larger than .05, say). One thing to note here is that added variables will never leave the model once they have been added. The second type of stepwise regression is **backward selection**; this method begins with a full model just like enter methods of regression. Next, it will find the most nonsignificant independent variable upon preset statistical criteria (e.g., $p > .05$) and take it out of the model. It will then find the next nonsignificant independent variable and delete it from the model, with this process continuing until there are no more nonsignificant independent variables in the pool. One thing to note here is that deleted variables from the model will never get back into the model. The last method is **stepwise selection**, and this method is a combination of the previous two. It begins with an empty model and finds the most significantly related independent variable to add it to the model, like the forward selection method. It will then find the next most significantly related independent variable and adds it to the model. This is where this method begins to differ from forward selection method. In the next step, you will reexamine the two previously entered independent variables to see if those two variables still remain significant for prediction. Since the addition or deletion of a variable can change the goodness of fit of the model, it is important to check for changes in the existing variables. You will continue to find the next significant independent variable based on preset statistical criteria if the two variables remain significant, but the nonsignificant variable will be eliminated from the model if the addition of second independent variable somehow makes the first added independent variable not significant. Unlike the forward and backward regression, a variable may be added or deleted from the model if the addition of other variables makes it significant or nonsignificant. The process continues until there is no significant variable left outside of the model. One thing to note is that this method relies on the statistical criteria the researcher sets and the computer makes the decisions in regards to the best prediction model. Therefore, it is possible that the fitted model created by this method may not actually be the best model for the data. In other words, a variable can be not included in the model just because it is not significant with defined statistical criteria in a given data, even if it is theoretically important.

So, the legitimate question to ask seems to be, which method do I use? You should consider the enter method as a rough examination procedure of the data, as nothing much can be done with a model built by forcing everything to be entered into the model simultaneously. Stepwise methods should be considered when a researcher wants to explore the data without preconceived ideas and see what the best prediction model is. If you are testing a theory or using what you have found in the literature to build the best model of prediction, hierarchical regression may be the choice. However, this method is only recommended when you have substantial knowledge about the variables in regards to what to control in the first block and what to test for significance in later blocks.

Now, let us go back to our example of systolic blood pressure with age and weight as predictors. To conduct multiple linear regression analysis in SPSS, you will go to Analyze > Regression > Linear as shown in **Figure 10-7**. In the Linear Regression dialogue box, you will move

Figure 10-7

Selecting multiple linear regression in SPSS.

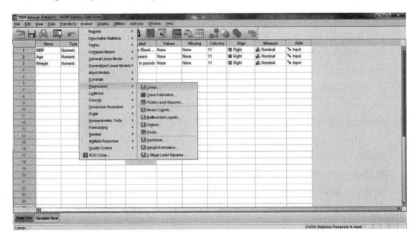

Figure 10-8

Defining variables in the Linear Regression box.

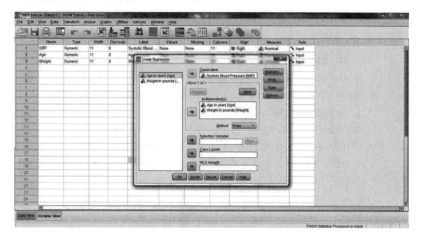

systolic blood pressure into "Dependent" and move age and weight into "Independent(s)" by clicking the corresponding arrow buttons in the middle as shown in **Figure 10-8**. For method, let us select "Forward" since we looked at "Enter" in the simple linear regression example.

There are some options that are useful in interpreting regression outputs, and they are "statistics," "plots," and "options." Under the "statistics" button, as shown in **Figure 10-9**, regression coefficient estimates

Figure 10-9

Statistics button in the regression box.

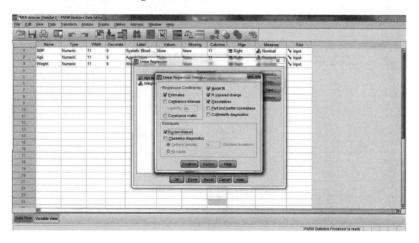

and model fit are checked by default because these two options will create important information about overall model fit and significance of each individual independent variable. However, let us check additional check boxes for the following:

- **R-squared change:** This option will examine the changes in R^2 with different stages of modeling for addition and deletion of a variable, so it will be helpful to address how much predictability each added variable adds to the model.
- **Descriptives:** It is always good to check descriptives to understand the data, so let us check this option as well.
- **Durbin–Watson:** This option will compute Durbin–Watson statistics to check the assumption of independence. You would want this statistic to be around $+2$ to avoid the violation.

In the Linear Regression Plots dialogue box, as shown in **Figure 10-10**, let us create a residual plot by moving "ZRESID" into Y and "ZPRED" into X to check the assumption of homogeneity of variance and linearity. You should not see any pattern in this plot if you were to meet those assumptions. In addition, you should check "Histogram" and "Normal probability plot" to check the assumption of normality.

In the Linear Regression Options dialogue box, as shown in **Figure 10-11**, you can play with probability criteria of entry and removal for

Figure 10-10

Linear Regression Plots dialogue box.

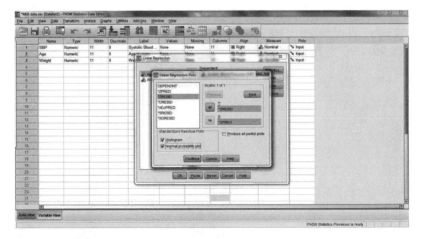

Figure 10-11

Linear Regression Options dialogue box.

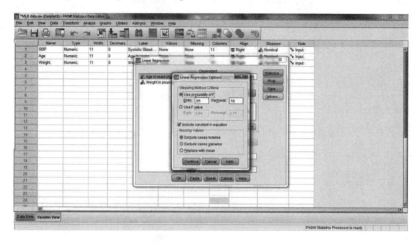

stepwise selection methods. The default is .05 for entry and .10 for removal, but you can make it more stringent or liberal.

Clicking "OK" will then produce the output of requested regression analysis. An example output is shown in **Table 10-5**.

Reporting Multiple Linear Regression

Reporting the results of multiple linear regressions is simply an extension of those in simple linear regression. It can be done in a table format and should include, at minimum, the unstandardized coefficients (B), standard error of unstandardized coefficients (B), standardized coefficients (β), and some overall statistics about the fitted model such as R^2. However, you will have additional rows representing additional variables with enter methods as compared to simple linear regression. Example reporting for our scenario, shown in **Table 10-6**, is for the forward method. Results indicate that both age and weight are significant predictor variables of systolic blood pressure with both sharing 98% of the variability in systolic blood pressure. However, age is the more important variable for prediction, as by itself it explains 95% of the total variability.

Table	
10-5	**Example Outputs of Multiple Linear Regression**

Descriptive Statistics

	Mean	Std. Deviation	N
Systolic blood pressure	150.09	13.627	11
Age in years	62.45	9.114	11
Weight in pounds	195.00	17.315	11

Correlations

		Systolic Blood Pressure	Age in Years	Weight in Pounds
Pearson correlation	Systolic blood pressure	1.000	.979	.971
	Age in years	.979	1.000	.946
	Weight in pounds	.971	.946	1.000
Sig. (1-tailed)	Systolic blood pressure		.000	.000
	Age in years	.000		.000
	Weight in pounds	.000	.000	
N	Systolic blood pressure	11	11	11
	Age in years	11	11	11
	Weight in pounds	11	11	11

Model Summary[b]

				Std. Error of the Estimate	Change Statistics					Durbin–Watson
Model	R	R- Square	Adjusted R-Square		R-Square Change	F Change	df1	df2	Sig. F Change	
1	.988[a]	.977	.971	2.318	.977	168.765	2	8	.000	1.927

[a] Predictors: (Constant), weight in pounds, age in years
[b] Dependent variable: Systolic blood pressure

(continued)

ANOVA[b]					
Model		**Sum of Squares**	**df**	**Mean Square**	**F**	**Sig.**
1	Regression	1813.916	2	906.958	168.765	.000[a]
	Residual	42.993	8	5.374		
	Total	1856.909	10			

[a] Predictors: (Constant), weight in pounds, age in years
[b] Dependent variable: Systolic blood pressure

Coefficients[a]						
		Unstandardized Coefficients		**Standardized Coefficients**		
Model		**B**	**Std. Error**	**Beta**	**t**	**Sig.**
1	(Constant)	30.994	11.944		2.595	.032
	Age in years	.861	.248	.576	3.470	.008
	Weight in pounds	.335	.131	.425	2.563	.034

[a] Dependent variable: Systolic blood pressure

Table 10-6	Example Reporting of Multiple Linear Regression Results		
	B	*SE (B)*	*β*
Step 1			
Constant	58.71	6.45	
Age in years	1.46	.10	.98[*]
Step 2			
Constant	20.99	11.94	
Age in years	.86	.25	.58[**]
Weight in pounds	.34	.13	.43[*]

Note: $R^2 = .95$ for step 1, $\Delta R^2 = .03$ for step 2 ($p < .05$).[*] $p < .05$. [**] $p < .01$.

LOGISTIC REGRESSION

Introduction

Logistic regression is multiple linear regressions with a categorical dependent variable and where independent variables can be either continuous or categorical. It can be **binary logistic regression** if a dependent variable is dichotomous with only two outcomes and **multinomial logistic regression** if a dependent variable is categorical with more than two outcomes. However, only binary logistic regression will be discussed in this chapter due to the extensive complexity of multinomial logistic regression.

Logistic regression can be used to predict group membership based on information collected from different independent variables. For example, one can use logistic regression to predict whether or not a patient will fail a surgery from knowledge about a patient's age, blood pressure, weight, and the number of days in the hospital. Or, using our previous example with per capita gross domestic product, we could predict life expectancy: long or short.

Doing and Interpreting Logistic Regression

To explain logistic regression, let us consider the data in the file, LR data.sav. There are three variables: age in years, weight in pounds, and surgery outcome. Our goal is to see if we can create a good prediction model for a surgery outcome using age and weight.

As always, the first step is to check whether the required assumptions are met. In fact, logistic regression violates many assumptions required by multiple linear regression due to the fact that the dependent variable is not continuous. Some of the assumptions to be met are:

- **Discrete dependent variable:** The dependent variable should be discrete or measured at the nominal level so that we predict group membership from independent variables.
- **Linearity between the logit of dependent variable and continuous independent variables:** As previously discussed, linearity assumptions for linear regression will be violated with logistic regression since the dependent variable is not continuous. Therefore,

we take the logit of dependent variable and examine its relationship with continuous independent variables to see if it is linear.

- **Independence:** The values of dependent variables are assumed to be independent, meaning that none of the values are from the same person.
- **No multicollinearity:** Like in linear regressions, having variables measuring the same thing can make the model complicated with not much gain in predictability. Therefore, we should examine for multicollinearity and remove one of the variables if it exists.

As with multiple linear regressions, you can choose between the enter method and the stepwise methods.

Overall Model Fit

Once the logistic model has been fitted to the data, we should examine how good the fitted model is for predicting group memberships. Logistic regression analysis will output -2 log-likelihood, Cox & Snell R^2, and Nagelkerke R^2 for the model summary. The statistic, -2 log-likelihood, represents a more desirable model when it is lower; the model with independent variable(s) should have lower -2 log-likelihood as compared to a constant-only model. Cox & Snell R^2 and Nagelkerke R^2 are indications of how well the model predicts group membership, and a higher figure represents a better model **(Figure 10-12)**.

Model Parameters

This part of output is where the significance of independent variables as predictors is shown, but the Wald test is used instead of a t-test to test significance of those independent variables. Interpretation should be the same as for the t-test. Under the following hypotheses:

H_0: $\beta_i = 0$ or independent variable does not do anything for prediction

H_a: $\beta_i \neq 0$ or independent variable is useful for prediction

the independent variable is said to be a good predictor when the associated p-value with Wald statistic of independent variable is less than alpha and not a good predictor when the associated p-value with Wald statistic of independent variable is larger than alpha.

Figure 10-12

Example model summary output.

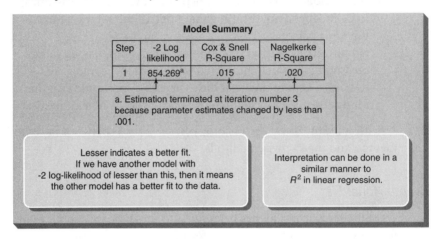

Model Summary			
Step	-2 Log likelihood	Cox & Snell R-Square	Nagelkerke R-Square
1	854.269[a]	.015	.020

a. Estimation terminated at iteration number 3 because parameter estimates changed by less than .001.

Lesser indicates a better fit. If we have another model with -2 log-likelihood of lesser than this, then it means the other model has a better fit to the data.

Interpretation can be done in a similar manner to R^2 in linear regression.

Odds Ratio: Exp (β)

Odds ratio is another important part of logistic regression outputs that tells us how much change in odds we would expect in a dependent variable following a unit change in an independent variable. Odds ratio can be defined as the ratio of odds of an event occurring for two groups. When the odds ratio is equal to 1, it means that the odds of an event occurring are the same for both groups. For our example, the odds of a patient dying are exactly the same for males and females. When the odds ratio is greater than 1, it means that the odds of an event occurring are greater for the male group (coded as 1) than for the female group (coded as 0). When the odds ratio is less than 1, it means that the odds of an event occurring are greater for the female group than for the male group. One thing to note about the odds ratio here is that corresponding confidence intervals should also be reported along with the odds ratio.

Predicted Probability and Classification Table

In SPSS, you can request predicted values of probability for classification, and it can help you understand how the classification is done. A classification table can also be obtained in SPSS, and this table will tell us how much correct classification we obtain with the currently fitted model. The higher the classification percentage is, the better the model is.

Figure 10-13

Selecting logistic regression in SPSS.

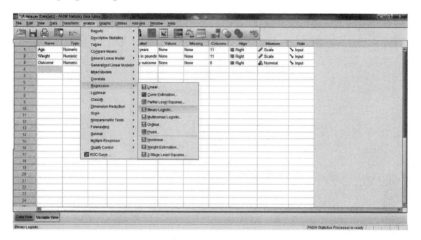

To conduct logistic regression in SPSS, you will go to Analyze > Regression > Binary Logistic, as shown in **Figure 10-13**. In the Logistic Regression dialogue box, you will select the variables you are interested in fitting a prediction line between and move an independent variable into "Independent(s)" and a dependent variable into "Dependent" by clicking the corresponding arrow buttons in the middle as shown in **Figure 10-14**.

Figure 10-14

Defining variables in SPSS.

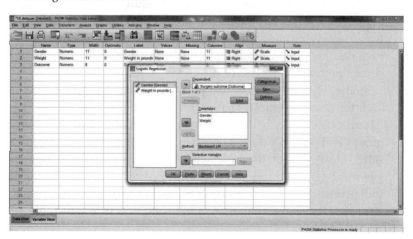

Figure 10-15

Categorical button in the regression dialogue box.

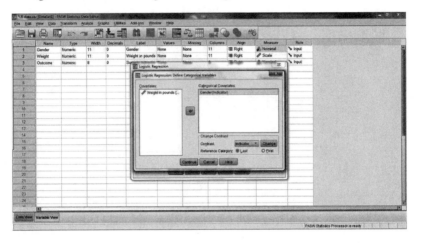

For method, we will select "Backward: LR" this time since we have discussed both the "Enter" and "Forward" procedures earlier in this chapter.

There are some options that are useful in interpreting logistic regression outputs, and they are "Categorical," "Save," and "Options." In the "Categorical" button, as shown in **Figure 10-15**, we define any categorical independent variables, if there are any. Gender is a categorical variable in our data, so we will select Gender and move it over to the "Categorical Covariates" window by clicking the arrow in the middle.

Under the "Save" button, as shown in **Figure 10-16**, you can request a predicted values probability and classification table. Let us check these two assumptions: that SPSS saves predicted probability values for each case and that it produces a classification table that we can check correct percentage of classification.

In the "Options" button, as shown in **Figure 10-17**, you can request additional useful options such as classification plots and CI for exp (β). Classification plots will show predicted probability of the observed group, and you will want to see two different symbols far from each other, ideally one on the far left end and the other on the far right end. CI for exp (β) will produce odds ratios and corresponding CI for each independent variable. Clicking "OK" will then produce the output of requested regression analysis. Example output is shown in **Table 10-7**.

Figure 10-16

Save button in the regression dialogue box.

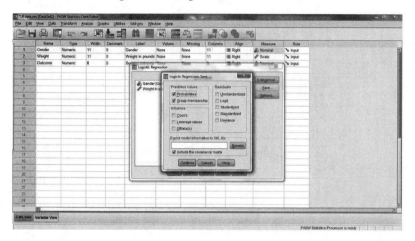

Reporting Logistic Regression

Just like other types of regression, the results can be clearly presented in a table and should include, at a minimum, coefficient B, standard error of B, odds ratios, and associated confidence interval.

Figure 10-17

Options button in the regression dialogue box.

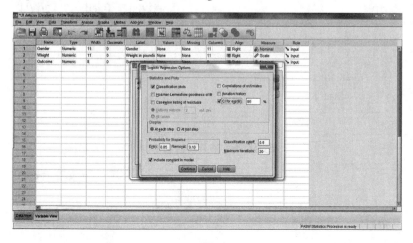

Table	
10-7	Example Output of Logistic Regression

Dependent Variable Encoding

Original Value	Internal Value
Survived	0
Dead	1

Categorical Variables Codings

			Parameter Coding
		Frequency	(1)
Gender	Male	9	1.000
	Female	11	.000

Block 0: Beginning Block

Classification Table[a,b]

			Predicted		
			Surgery Outcome		Percentage
Observed			Survived	Dead	Correct
Step 0	Surgery outcome	Survived	12	0	100.0
		Dead	8	0	.0
	Overall percentage				60.0

[a] Constant is included in the model.
[b] The cut value is .500.

Variables in the Equation

		B	S.E.	Wald	df	Sig.	Exp(B)
Step 0	Constant	−.405	.456	.789	1	.374	.667

(continues)

Variables Not in the Equation

			Score	df	Sig.
Step 0	Variables	Gender(1)	.135	1	.714
		Weight	7.473	1	.006
	Overall statistics		81740	2	.013

Block 1: Method = Backward Stepwise (Likelihood Ratio)

Omnibus Tests of Model Coefficients

		Chi-Square	df	Sig.
Step 1	Step	10.010	2	.007
	Block	10.010	2	.007
	Model	10.010	2	.007
Step 2[a]	Step	−1.371	1	.242
	Block	8.639	1	.003
	Model	8.639	1	.003

[a] A negative chi-square value indicates that the chi-square value has decreased from the previous step.

Model Summary

Step	−2 Log Likelihood	Cox & Snell R-Square	Nagelkerke R-Square
1	16.911[a]	.394	.532
2	18.281[a]	.351	.474

[a] Estimation terminated at iteration number 5 because parameter estimates changed by less than .001.

Classification Table[a]

			Predicted		
			Surgery Outcome		Percentage
Observed			Survived	Dead	Correct
Step 1	Surgery outcome	Survived	11	1	91.7
		Dead	2	6	75.0
	Overall percentage				85.0
Step 2	Surgery outcome	Survived	11	1	91.7
		Dead	2	6	75.0
	Overall percentage				85.0

[a] The cut value is .500.

(continues)

Table	
10-7	Continued

Variables in the Equation

		B	S.E.	Wald	df	Sig.	Exp(B)	95% CI for Exp(B) Lower	Upper
Step 1[a]	Gender(1)	1.450	1.304	1.236	1	.266	4.263	.331	54.925
	Weight	.100	.041	5.906	1	.015	1.105	1.019	1.198
	Constant	−20.504	8.245	6.184	1	.013	.000		
Step 2[a]	Weight	.092	.041	5.037	1	.025	1.096	1.012	1.187
	Constant	−18.267	8.000	5.214	1	.022	.000		

Model If Term Removed

	Variable	Model Log Likelihood	Change in −2 Log Likelihood	df	Sig. of the Change
Step 1	Gender	−9.141	1.371	1	.242
	Weight	−13.393	9.875	1	.002
Step 2	Weight	−13.460	8.639	1	.003

Variables Not in the Equation

			Score	df	Sig.
Step 2[a]	Variables	Gender(1)	1.325	1	.250
	Overall statistics		1.325	1	.250

[a] Variable(s) removed on step 2: Gender.

(continues)

```
Step number: 1

observed Groups and Predicted Probabilities

        4 +                                                                              +
          I                                                                              I
          I                                                                              I
          I                                                                              I
F       3 +                                                                              +
R         I                                                                              I
E         I                                                                              I
Q         I                                                                              I
U       2 +               S                                                              +
E         I               S                                                              I
N         I               S                                                              I
C         I               S                                                              I
Y       1 +   SSS  SD   S S   S S S   S        D              D    D        D   S D  DD   +
          I   SSS  SD   S S   S S S   S        D              D    D        D   S D  DD   I
          I   SSS  SD   S S   S S S   S        D              D    D        D   S D  DD   I
          I   SSS  SD   S S   S S S   S        D              D    D        D   S D  DD   I
Predicted ----+-----+-----+-----+-----+-----+-----+-----+-----+-----+-----
Prob:     0     .1      .2      .3      .4      .5      .6      .7      .8      .9      1
Group:   SSSSSSSSSSSSSSSSSSSSSSSSSSSSSSSSSSSSSSSSSSSSSSSSDDDDDDDDDDDDDDDDDDDDDDDDDDDDDDDDDDDDDDDDDDDDDDD

          Predicted Probability is of Membership for Dead
          The Cut Value is .50
          Symbols: S - Survived
                   D - Dead
          Each Symbol Represents .25 Cases.
```

```
Step number: 2

observed Groups and Predicted Probabilities

        4 +                                                                              +
          I                                                                              I
          I                                                                              I
          I                                                                              I
F       3 +                                                                              +
R         I                                                                              I
E         I                                                                              I
Q         I                                                                              I
U       2 +                     S                                                        +
E         I                     S                                                        I
N         I                     S                                                        I
C         I                     S                                                        I
Y       1 +  S S S  S S S   SD       S       S       S      D   D D          D    D       D  S   D   +
          I  S S S  S S S   SD       S       S       S      D   D D          D    D       D  S   D   I
          I  S S S  S S S   SD       S       S       S      D   D D          D    D       D  S   D   I
          I  S S S  S S S   SD       S       S       S      D   D D          D    D       D  S   D   I
Predicted ----+-----+-----+-----+-----+-----+-----+-----+-----+-----+-----
Prob:     0     .1      .2      .3      .4      .5      .6      .7      .8      .9      1
Group:   SSSSSSSSSSSSSSSSSSSSSSSSSSSSSSSSSSSSSSSSSSSSSSSSDDDDDDDDDDDDDDDDDDDDDDDDDDDDDDDDDDDDDDDDDDDDDDD

          Predicted Probability is of Membership for Dead
          The Cut Value is .50
          Symbols: S - Survived
                   D - Dead
          Each Symbol Represents .25 Cases.
```

Table				
10-8	**Example Reporting of Logistic Regression Results**			
			95% CI for Odds Ratio	
	B (SE)	**Lower**	**Odds Ratio**	**Upper**
Step 1				
Gender	1.45 (1.30)	.33	4.26	54.93
Weight	.10 (.04)	1.02	1.11	1.20
Constant	−20.50 (8.25)		.00	
Step 2				
Weight	.92 (.04)	1.10	2.00	1.19
Constant	−18.27 (8.00)		.00	

Example reporting for logistics regression results is shown in **Table 10-8**. Our example results indicate that only weight is a significant predictor variable of surgery outcome and the model with only gender included produces a correct classification of 85%. Odds ratio for weight tells us that the probability of a patient failing surgery increases as his/her weight increases, since the corresponding odds ratio is greater than 1.

SUMMARY

Regression analysis builds on results from correlation coefficients to predict one variable from the other. Simple linear regression is used when we need to predict a single continuous dependent variable using a single continuous independent variable. In order to do simple linear regression, you will first draw and examine a scatterplot of the data and visually check the strength of the linear relationship between variables. Second, you will compute the correlation coefficients as a numerical verification of what you saw in a scatterplot if the relationship in the plot appears relatively strong. Finally, you will try to fit the best line of prediction through regression analysis if the correlation coefficient still comes out to be significant.

Multiple linear regression is a natural extension of simple linear regression where more than one independent variable is used to predict a continuous dependent variable. Prediction models can be fitted using one of the three methods: enter, hierarchical, and stepwise; the decision of which to use should be made based on whether you want to explore the data or to test a theory from the literature. The best prediction model is often times the one that has fewer predictor variables, but still explains a substantial variability in a dependent variable.

Logistic regression is essentially multiple linear regressions with a discrete dependent variable; therefore, the goal is to predict group membership, not the value of the dependent variable. Similar model selection methods as with multiple linear regressions can be used in logistic regression, and the goal is to find the best prediction model with fewer predictor variables.

Critical Thinking Questions

1. Discuss the importance of prediction in research and clinical practice.
2. Let's say you want to know if the number of days hospitalized is a significant predictor of accidental falls among patients. How would you set up a simple linear regression or logistic regression to test this hypothesis?
3. Which stepwise approach to multiple linear regression would be the best when testing a harm reduction theory for predicting smoking cessation?
4. In regression analyses, R^2 seems to provide important information in regard to model predictability. Let us assume that a researcher obtained R^2 of 35% in a study, which seems to be higher than the results from similar types of research in the literature. How should the researcher report these results in terms of contribution to the literature?
5. Use the data file *SBP.sav* (found on the Student Companion Website using the access code card from the front of this text) and run a simple linear regression analysis. Report the findings in APA format. Discuss how well age predicts systolic blood pressure (SBP).
6. In the following case study, identify the predictor and dependent variables and the type of regression analysis used. What conclusion may be made about the strength of predictions resulting from the analysis?

Case Study

Cox, J. (2011). Predictors of pressure ulcers in adult critical care patients. *American Journal of Critical Care, 20*(5), 364–374.

Objective: To determine which risk factors are most predictive of pressure ulcers in adult critical care patients. Risk factors investigated included total score on the Braden Scale, mobility, activity, sensory perception, moisture, friction/shear, nutrition, age, blood pressure, length of stay in the intensive care unit, score on the Acute Physiology and Chronic Health Evaluation II, vasopressor administration, and comorbid conditions.

Methods: A retrospective, correlational design was used to examine 347 patients admitted to a medical-surgical intensive care unit from October 2008 through May 2009.

Results: According to logistic regression analyses, age, length of stay, mobility, friction/shear, norepinephrine infusion, and cardiovascular disease explained a major part of the variance in pressure ulcers.

Logistic regression ($n = 347$)

Variable	B	Standard Error	Wald	P	Exp(B)	95% Confidence Interval
Age	0.033	0.015	4.725	.03	1.033	1.003 to 1.064
Hours in intensive care unit	0.008	0.002	21.996	< .001	1.008	1.005 to 1.011
Cardiovascular disease	1.082	0.401	7.288	.007	2.952	1.3 to 6.4
Mobility	−0.823	0.398	4.262	.04	0.439	0.210 to 0.95
Constant	−7.049	2.857	6.087	.01	0.001	

Nagelkerke $R^2 = 0.512$.
Hosmer and Lemeshow test: $\chi^2 = 6.993$, $df = 8$, $P = .54$.

Logistic regression (n = 327), subsample of all patients excluding patients with stage I pressure ulcers

Variable	B	Standard Error	Wald	P	Exp(B)	95% Confidence Interval
Hours in intensive care unit	0.008	0.002	18.063	< .001	1.008	1.004 to 1.012
Cardiovascular disease	1.218	0.519	5.510	.02	3.380	1.223 to 9.347
Friction/shear	1.743	0.709	6.039	.01	5.715	1.423 to 22.95
Norepinephrine	0.017	0.008	4.223	.04	1.017	1.001 to 1.033
Constant	−10.512	3.779	7.737	.005	0.000	

Nagelkerke R^2 = 0.569.
Hosmer and Lemeshow test: χ^2 = 5.836, df = 8, P = .67.

Self-Quiz www

1. True or false: Predicting the variance on a dependent variable based on variation on the independent variable is an important step toward controlling health-related phenomena.
2. True or false: It is still important to run a regression analysis even when the relationship is not found to be significant with a scatterplot and correlation coefficient.
3. A regression analysis found a prediction line for systolic blood pressure with age to be $y = 100 + .25 \times X$. What would be the predicted systolic blood pressure when a selected patient is 42 years old?
4. True or false: If a researcher finds an R-square of .55, this means that 55% of the variance on the dependent variable can be explained by the independent variable.

REFERENCES

Aggar, C., Ronaldson, S., & Cameron, I. D. (2010). Reactions to caregiving of frail, older persons predict depression. *International Journal of Mental Health Nursing, 19*, 409–415.

Cengage Learning. (2010). Systolic blood pressure data: Data for multiple linear regression [Data file]. Retrieved from http://college.cengage.com/ mathematics/brase/understandable_statistics/7e/students/datasets/mlr/ frames/frame.html

Cox, J. (2011). Predictors of pressure ulcers in adult critical care patients. *American Journal of Critical Care, 20*(5), 364–374.

Durbin, J., & Watson, G. S. (1951). Testing for serial correlation in least squares regression II. *Biometrika, 38*(1–2), 159–178.

11

Tests for Comparing Group Means: Part I

Learning Objectives

The principal goal of this chapter is to explain the purpose of statistical tests of differences between means (difference tests), when they may be used, and how to interpret the results. This chapter will prepare you to:

- Understand approaches to difference testing to answer a proposed research question
- Evaluate assumptions of difference tests
- Distinguish an independent sample difference test from a dependent sample difference test
- Understand the purpose of multiple comparison testing
- Distinguish how the number of groups influences the choice of statistical test of difference
- Correctly report the findings of difference tests in APA style
- Understand how tests of differences are used in evidence-based practice

Key Terms

Analysis of variance (ANOVA)

Bonferroni correction

Dependent group

F-statistic

Independent group

Omega squared

Orthogonal planned contrasts

Post hoc tests

t-test

Univariate

INTRODUCTION

Tests of differences of means are used to make comparisons. In health-care research, we are often interested in comparing treatments to determine which is more effective. Such analyses may be found in descriptive comparative studies or experimental designs. For example, in a descriptive comparative study, we may ask how cancer incidence varies depending on sex or gender. To be more specific, we might ask, "Does the mean number of new cases of lung cancer each year differ by sex?" Descriptive comparative studies help to explain phenomena that occur naturally without the researcher influencing any variables.

Testing the statistical significance between means is also applied to experimental questions. Experimental designs are highly controlled so that the researcher can determine the effect of the independent variable on the dependent variable. We may want to know what treatment or intervention produces the best outcome, such as "On average, which wound care treatment reduces healing time the most?" In both of our examples, we must be able to calculate a mean value for the dependent variable in order to make comparisons between means; here, the average number of new cases of lung cancer each year and the average time for wound healing, respectively. These tests require that dependent variables be continuous or measured at the interval or ratio level. In this chapter, we will discuss a number of statistical tests that compare group means of a continuous variable(s).

Case Study

Saban, K. L., Smith, B. M., Collins, E. G., & Bender Pape, T. L. (2011). Sex differences in perceived life satisfaction and functional status one year after severe traumatic brain injury. *Journal of Women's Health, 20*(2), 179–186. doi: 10.1089=jwh.2010.2334

Dr. Karen Saban and colleagues (2011) noted that traumatic brain injury is the most common injury experienced by people living in the United States, but that little is known about the variables that influence neurological outcomes. In particular, Saban et al. suggest that hormones, such as estrogen and progesterone, which are shown to have protective effects in animals, may positively influence neurological outcomes in humans. To test this hypothesis, the researchers designed a descriptive comparative study examining the differences between outcomes of traumatic brain injury in men and women. In other words, Saban et al. wanted to know if there are differences between the two sexes on functional status, rehabilitation, and injury severity in brain-injured patients. The researchers used independent t-tests to analyze data from 297 participants ($n = 80$ women and $n = 213$ men). Saban et al. did find a statistically significant difference on quality of life at 1 year, with women having lower scores than men. Saban and colleagues concluded from this study that sex might influence patient outcomes following traumatic brain injury, but that additional research is needed to determine the role of hormones in interventions.

Saban et al.'s study is a good example of comparing differences between groups—in this case, between men and women. We can begin now to think of other examples of group comparisons: between age groups, race or ethnicity, experimental and control groups, or even comparisons from the same group, all women, but at different times. We also are not limited to comparing two groups; group comparisons can be made among three or more groups.

CHOOSING THE RIGHT STATISTICAL TEST

Choosing the right statistical test depends upon the proposed research questions and consideration of factors such as the number of groups that will be compared. In group comparisons, the independent variable is often called the grouping variable. In the Saban et al. case study, the grouping variable was sex and participants were either men or women. It is easy to confuse groups with variables. For example, if the independent variable was ethnicity (one independent variable) and participants were white, black, or Asian (three groups), some might mistakenly think that there are three independent variables instead of a single grouping variable—ethnicity—with three groups. It is standard practice as you are designing research or reading research reports to ask yourself, "What are the independent and dependent variables in this study?"

Another important consideration is whether the groups are independent or dependent, which is often times confusing. Therefore, we recommend that you pay special attention to the discussion of independence, to be found in a later section.

ONE-SAMPLE *t*-TEST

The *t*-**test** is used in the simplest situation, where two means are being compared, and a one-sample *t*-test is the simplest *t*-test. A one-sample *t*-test compares the mean score of a sample on a continuous dependent variable to a known value, which is a population mean. For example, say we take a sample of students from the university and compare their mean IQ to a known average IQ for the university. If we want to find out whether a sample mean IQ differs from the average university IQ, a one-sample *t*-test will give us the answer.

There are three assumptions to be met for one sample *t*-test. First, we should know the population mean, since the sample mean will be compared to it. Second, the sample should be randomly selected from the population and the subjects within the sample should be independent of each other (no participant will be sampled more than once). Lastly, the dependent variable should be continuous and normally distributed.

Doing and Interpreting a One-Sample *t*-Test

As with all hypotheses testing, we need to first set up the hypotheses:

H_0: There is no significant difference between the sample mean and a known population mean.

H_a: There is a significant difference between the sample mean and a known population mean.

or

$$H_0: \mu = 120$$
$$H_a: \mu \neq 120$$

and determine a level of significance from among .10, .05, .01, and .001.

The test statistic for a one-sample *t*-test can be found by using the following formula:

$$t = \frac{\bar{x} - \mu}{\dfrac{s}{\sqrt{n}}}$$

where $\bar{x}$ is the sample mean, μ is the population mean, s is the sample standard deviation, and n is the sample size. Then, the *p*-value associated with the computed statistic is compared with alpha and the decision is made (i.e., the null hypothesis is rejected when the *p*-value associated with the computed statistic is smaller than the alpha or not rejected when the *p*-value associated with the computed statistic is larger than the alpha).

To conduct a one-sample *t*-test in SPSS, you will go to Analyze > Compare means > One-sample *t*-test as shown in **Figure 11-1**, in

Figure 11-1

Selecting a one-sample *t*-test in SPSS.

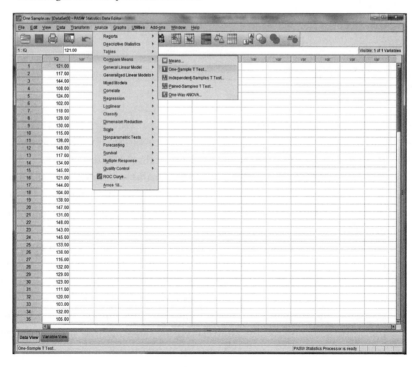

Figure 11-2

Defining variables in a one-sample *t*-test in SPSS.

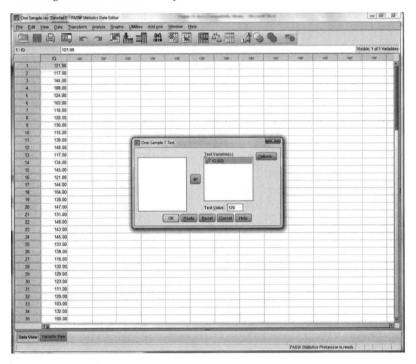

this case using IQ measurements from a sample of nursing students. In the One-Sample *t*-Test dialogue box, you will move IQ into "Test variable(s)" by clicking on the arrow buttons in the middle and typing in a known population mean into "Test value" (**Figure 11-2**).

In the Option menu, the default for confidence interval percentage is 95%, but you can change it to a different percentage, such as 90% or 99%, if you want to use a level of significance other than .05. This menu also gives you options for dealing with missing values. The default is to "exclude cases by analysis," which excludes cases if they have missing values on variables in the current analysis. The other option is to "exclude cases listwise;" this option deletes cases that have any missing values on any variables, whether in the current analysis or a prior one. If cases have even one missing value on a single variable, they will be excluded from the entire analysis, and the analysis is done only on those with complete values. Clicking "OK" will then produce the output of requested regression analysis. The example output is shown in **Table 11-1**.

Table	
11-1	Example Output of a One-Sample *t*-Test

One-Sample Statistics

	N	Mean	Std. Deviation	Std. Error Mean
IQ	100	125.1100 *AVG*	14.93751	1.49375

One-Sample Test

Test Value = 120

	t-statistic t	df	*(p-value)* Sig. (2-tailed)	Mean Difference	95% Confidence Interval of the Difference Lower	Upper
IQ	3.421	99	.001	5.11000	2.1461	8.0739

You will see that the average IQ of the sample was 125.11 and the *t*-statistic and corresponding *p*-value are 3.421 and .001, respectively. Since the *p*-value is less than our alpha of .05, the null hypothesis is rejected, and we determine that the average IQ of this sample of nursing students is not equal to 120. In fact, they have higher IQ by 5.11 units.

Reporting One-Sample *t*-Test Results

When reporting one-sample *t*-test results, you should report the size of the *t*-statistics and associated *p*-value and also report means and standard error so that the readers will know how the sample statistic is different from the known population parameter. Cohen's *d*, a type of effect size as discussed in Chapter 7, can also be computed and reported. Results of the *t*-test for our example for IQ variable could be reported like this:

- Nursing students of the current cohort at ABC University had significantly higher IQ scores ($M = 125.11$, $SE = 1.49$) than did ABC University students in general, $t(99) = 3.42$, $p < .001$, $d = .34$.

R INDEPENDENT GROUPS

tests are used when there are two **independent groups**
ιυ υε ωmpared on their means. By "independent," we mean that the
subjects in one group cannot also be members of the other group. The
t-statistic is computed by dividing the difference between means by
an estimate of the standard error of the difference between those two
independent sample means. A large deviation between means suggests that the samples from the population differ a lot, while a small
deviation between means suggests that samples from the population
are more similar.

Rationale

The basis for using the t-test is that the standard error is used as a gauge
of the variability between sample means. When the standard error is
large, we will observe large differences in sample means, and we will
observe small differences in sample means when the standard error is
small. For example, in experimental studies, where we are often comparing treatments or interventions, we reject the null hypothesis when
sample means are statistically different because of the manipulation
of the independent variable by a researcher. Otherwise, the difference
between sample means is occurring by chance only.

Assumptions

The following parametric assumptions should be met before the independent samples t-test is performed.

- The sampling distribution should be normal (i.e., the dependent variable should be normally distributed)
- The data should be measured at the interval level, at least (i.e.,
  continuous measurement)
- Variances in the groups being compared should be about the same
- Measurements should be independent (i.e., subjects in these
  two groups should not overlap).

Refer to Chapter 8 for the details about how to check these assumptions.

Doing and Interpreting Independent Samples *t*-Test

First, we need to set up hypotheses:

H_0: There is no significant difference between group 1 mean and group 2 mean.

H_a: There is a significant difference between group 1 mean and group 2 mean.

or

$$H_0: \mu_1 = \mu_2$$
$$H_a: \mu_1 \neq \mu_2$$

and choose the level of significance from among .10, .05, .01, and .001.

The test statistic for independent samples *t*-test can be found by using one of the following formulas:

$$t = \frac{\bar{x}_1 - \bar{x}_2}{\sqrt{\dfrac{S_1^2}{N_1} + \dfrac{S_2^2}{N_2}}} \text{ when sample sizes are equal}$$

$$t = \frac{\bar{x}_1 - \bar{x}_2}{\sqrt{S_p^2\left(\dfrac{1}{n_1} + \dfrac{1}{n_2}\right)}} \text{ when sample sizes are not equal}$$

where

$$S_p^2 = \frac{(n_1 - 1)S_1^2 + (n_2 - 1)S_2^2}{n_1 + n_2 - 2}$$

Once the statistic is computed, the associated *p*-value is compared with alpha and the decision is made (i.e., the null hypothesis is rejected when the *p*-value associated with the computed statistic is smaller than the alpha or not rejected when the *p*-value associated with the computed statistic is larger than the alpha).

To conduct an independent samples *t*-test in SPSS, you will go to Analyze > Compare means >Independent samples *t*-test as shown in **Figure 11-3** (the data shown in the figure are the number of beds in nursing homes in the states of Illinois and Ohio). In the Independent Samples *t*-Test dialogue box, you will move a dependent variable, "NB," into "Test variable(s)" and the independent variable, "State," into "Grouping variable" by clicking the corresponding

Figure 11-3

Selecting an independent samples *t*-test in SPSS.

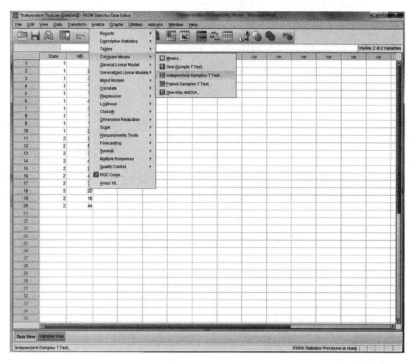

arrow buttons in the middle, as seen in **Figure 11-4**. You will notice that the "OK" button is not active because we have not defined our two groups. As you see in **Figure 11-5**, we have defined the coding of 1 for Illinois and 2 for Ohio. Click on the "Define Groups" button and assign 1 for group 1 and 2 for group 2 (**Figure 11-6**). Clicking "Continue" and then "OK" will produce the output of the requested analysis. The example output is shown in **Table 11-2**.

You will see that the average number of nursing home beds per nursing home in the state of Illinois is 23.8, and that in the state of Ohio the average is 34.2. We see that there is about a 10-bed difference between the two states; the question is whether this difference of 10 beds is statistically significant. Recall one of the assumptions was that the variability of the two groups is about the same. Independent

Figure 11-4

Defining variables in an independent samples *t*-test in SPSS.

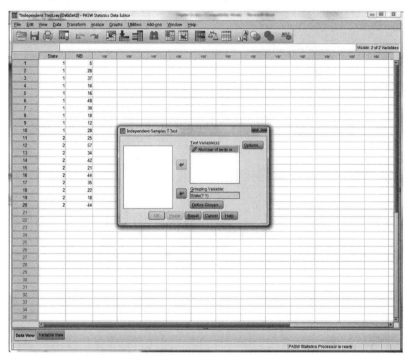

samples *t*-test outputs include the results of a test, Levene's test, which checks this assumption under the following hypotheses:

H_0: Variances of the two groups are equal.

H_a: Variances of the two groups are not equal.

or

$$H_0: \sigma_1^2 = \sigma_2^2$$
$$H_a: \sigma_1^2 \neq \sigma_2^2$$

The assumption of equal variance is said to be violated when the *p*-value is smaller than a prespecified alpha (i.e., the result is significant) and the assumption is said to be not violated otherwise (i.e., the result is not significant). You should interpret the results of an independent

Figure 11-5

Coding scheme for "State" variable.

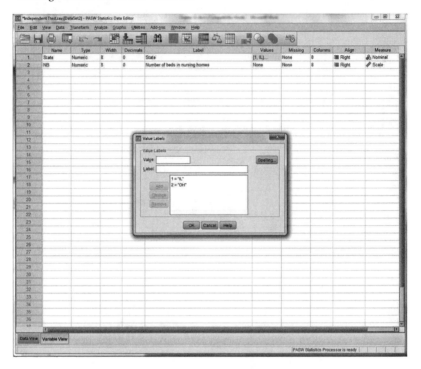

samples *t*-test according to this result. If Levene's test is not significant, you should interpret the first row of the output, "Equal variances assumed," and the second row of the output, "Equal variances not assumed." In our example, the assumption of equal variances is not violated, so we will interpret the "Equal variances assumed" row of the output. The computed *t*-statistic and corresponding *p*-value are -1.824 and $.085$, respectively. Since the *p*-value is larger than our alpha of $.05$, the null hypothesis is not rejected and it is determined that the average number of beds in Illinois and Ohio nursing homes is said to be roughly the same.

Reporting Independent Samples *t*-Test Results

When reporting independent samples *t*-test results, you should report the size of the *t*-statistic and associated *p*-value and also report means

Figure 11-6

Defining groups in an independent samples *t*-test in SPSS.

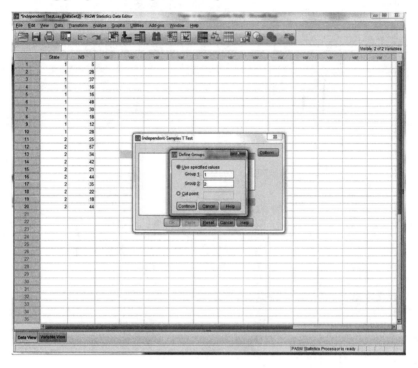

and standard error so that the readers will know how the two sample means differ. Another type of effect size, *r*, as discussed in Chapter 7, can be computed with the following equation

$$r = \sqrt{\frac{t^2}{t^2 + df}}$$

and reported for the independent sample *t*-test. The following is a sample report for our example:

- On average, the number of beds in Illinois nursing homes ($M = 23.8$, $SE = 4.06$) was not significantly different from the number of beds in Ohio nursing homes ($M = 34.2$, $SE = 4.01$), $t(18) = -1.83$, $p = .085$, $r = .40$.

Table 11-2 Example Output of an Independent Samples *t*-Test in SPSS

Group Statistics

	State	N	Mean	Std. Deviation	Std. Error Mean
Number of beds in nursing homes	IL	10	23.80	12.831	~~4.057~~
	OH	10	34.20	12.665	~~4.005~~

Independent Samples Test

	Levene's Test for Equality of Variances		*t*-Test for Equality of Means					95% Confidence Interval of the Difference	
	F	Sig.	t	df	Sig. (2-tailed)	Mean Difference	Std. Error Difference	Lower	Upper
Number of beds in nursing homes									
Equal variances assumed	.004	.947	−1.824	18	.085	−10.400	5.701	−22.378	1.578
Equal variances not assumed			−1.824	17.997	.085	−10.400	5.701	−22.378	1.578

(handwritten annotations: "p value" pointing to −1.824 and to .085)

t-TEST FOR DEPENDENT GROUP

(Paired)

The dependent samples t-test is used when the me
dependent variable are paired. By dependent samp
are dealing with a single group of participants, an   ...es to
one set of measurements influences their response. to another. There
are two ways that measurements can be paired. First, one sample can be
measured twice, such as when the systolic blood pressure of a group of
patients was measured before and after they received an antihypertensive drug. Second, two different data sets can be paired, such as when
a group of survey participants gives ratings of two different products
at the same time. The statistic is computed in the same way as in the
independent samples t-test, in that the difference between the means is
divided by some form of the standard error. Measurement will differ a
lot if there is a large deviation between means, and measurements will
not differ much if there is small deviation between means. The same
rationale discussed previously for the independent samples t-test still
applies for the dependent samples t-test.

Assumptions

As measurements will not be independent, we cannot assume that the
last two assumptions of the independent t-test, which are the assumptions of equal variance and independent measurements, are valid.
However, the normality of sampling distribution and data being measured at the interval level still apply.

One thing to note about the two assumptions for a dependent
samples t-test is that what has to be measured at least at the interval
level and to be normally distributed are not the measurements themselves. It is, in fact, the difference between the two sets of measurements. For example, we need to check the level of measurement and
normality of the difference between systolic blood pressure measurements before and after receiving an antihypertensive drug, not before
and after measurements themselves. Therefore, the first task is to
calculate the difference between the measurements for each case in
the data set, and then you should examine the level of measurements
and the normality of it.

Doing and Interpreting Dependent Samples *t*-Test

First, we need to set up hypotheses:

H_0: There is no significant difference between before measurements and after measurements.

H_a: There is a significant difference between before measurements and after measurements.

or

$$H_0: \mu_B = \mu_A$$
$$H_a: \mu_B \neq \mu_A$$

and choose the level of significance from among .10, .05, .01, and .001.

The test statistic for dependent samples *t*-test can be found by the following equation:

$$t = \frac{\overline{D} - \mu_D}{\dfrac{S_D}{\sqrt{N}}}$$

where $\overline{D}$ is the mean difference between sample measurements, μ_D is the hypothesized mean difference between population measurements, and S_D is the standard error of the difference. Once the statistic is computed, the associated *p*-value is then compared with alpha, and the decision is made (i.e., the null hypothesis is rejected when the *p*-value associated with the computed statistic is smaller than the alpha or not rejected when the *p*-value associated with the computed statistic is larger than the alpha).

To conduct a dependent samples *t*-test in SPSS, you will go to Analyze > Compare means > Paired samples *t*-test as shown in **Figure 11-7**. The data shown in this figure are sodium content levels in a sample of patients both before and after a new diet. In the Paired Samples *t*-Test dialogue box, then you will move the variables to be paired into "Paired Variables," in order, by clicking the corresponding arrow buttons in the middle as shown in **Figure 11-8**. Clicking "OK" will then produce the output of the requested analysis. An example output is shown in **Table 11-3**.

You will see that the average sodium content level before the new diet is 145.6 units and the average sodium content level after a new diet is 139.0 units. We see that there is a difference of 6.6 in sodium content

Figure 11-7

Selecting a dependent samples *t*-test in SPSS.

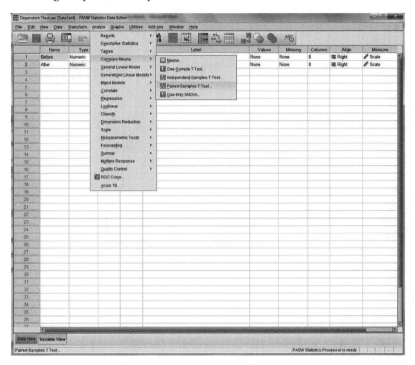

level between the before and after; the question now is whether or not this difference of 6.6 units of sodium is statistically significant. The second section in Table 11-3 shows that the measurements are significantly correlated, with a correlation coefficient of .88 and its associated *p*-value of .001. The computed *t*-statistic and corresponding *p*-value are −5.44 and .000, respectively. Since the *p*-value is less than our alpha of .05, the null hypothesis is rejected, and it is determined that the average sodium content level before a new diet is significantly higher than the one measured after a new diet.

Reporting Dependent Samples *t*-Test

When reporting dependent samples *t*-test results, you should report the size of *t*-statistic and associated *p* value and also report means and

Figure 11-8

Defining variables in a dependent samples *t*-test in SPSS.

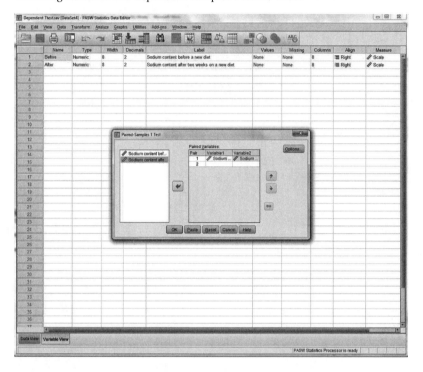

standard error so that the readers will know how the sample statistic is different from the known population parameter. As discussed previously for the independent samples *t*-test, *r* can be computed and reported for the dependent sample *t*-test. The following is a sample report of our example:

- On average, the sodium content level after a new diet ($M = 145.6$, $SE = 2.45$) was significantly lower than that before a new diet ($M = 139.0$, $SE = 2.41$), $t(9) = 5.44$, $p = .001$, $r = .88$.

ONE-WAY ANALYSIS OF VARIANCE (ANOVA)

The independent *t*-test allows us to compare the means of two independent groups and to make decisions on whether or not they are significantly different. What if we have more than two groups we want

Table

11-3 Example Output of a Dependent Samples *t*-Test in SPSS

Paired Samples Statistics

	Mean	N	Std. Deviation	Std. Error Mean
Pair 1 Sodium content before a new diet	145.6000	10	7.76316	2.45493
Sodium content after 2 weeks on a new diet	139.0000	10	7.63035	2.41293

Paired Samples Correlations

	N	Correlation	Sig.
Pair 1 Sodium content before a new diet and sodium content after 2 weeks on a new diet	10	.876	.001

Paired Samples Test

	Paired Differences					t	df	Sig. (2-tailed)
				95% Confidence Interval of the Difference				
	Mean	Std. Deviation	Std. Error Mean	Lower	Upper			
Pair 1 Sodium content before a new diet and sodium content after 2 weeks on a new diet	6.60000	3.83551	1.21289	3.85624	9.34376	5.442	9	.000

to compare? For example, let us assume that a nurse researcher is interested in testing the effectiveness of a newly developed diet using three groups: a placebo group, an existing diet group, and a new diet group. Because the independent t-test is only designed to test two group means, the simultaneous comparison of these three groups is not possible. You may be thinking that it is possible to conduct three independent samples t-tests by comparing the following pairs: placebo–existing diet, placebo–new diet, and existing diet–new diet. However, there is an increased risk of type I error as we conduct multiple tests this way, and this increased risk gets worse as the number of tests increases (i.e., the actual risk of type I error will be greater than the prespecified alpha as the number of tests increases). This will be true for any set of statistical tests.

For any given set of statistical tests, the inflated type I error will be:

$$\alpha_{Inflated} = 1 - (1 - \alpha_{prespecified})^n$$

where $\alpha_{Inflated}$ is the type I error inflated after conducting multiple tests, $\alpha_{prespecified}$ is the prespecified/desired type I error, and n is the number of tests. As you can see, the risk of type I error will be inflated as more tests are conducted. For example, if you run three tests, each at a type I error of .05, the type I error is inflated to

$$\alpha_{Inflated} = 1 - (1 - .05)^3 = .1426$$

and running five tests will inflate the type I error to

$$\alpha_{Inflated} = 1 - (1 - .05)^5 = .2262$$

So, what do .1426 and .2262 mean? They mean that you have a higher probability of committing a type I error by conducting multiple tests (i.e., you will be more prone to falsely reject the null hypothesis when it is actually true). Therefore, you should control for an inflated type I error somehow so that you will not have a higher risk of making a type I error than you desired.

A common remedy to adjust for type I error inflation is the **Bonferroni correction**. This method adjusts the type I error rate per test so that the type I error for multiple tests remains at the prespecified type I error. The correction is made by dividing the preselected alpha by the number of tests. For example, you will compare the computed p-value against

$$\alpha' = \frac{\alpha}{n} = \frac{0.05}{5} = .01$$

if you were to use $\alpha = .05$ for five separate tests. Let us assume that the *p*-value of one of the five tests came out to be .02. It will be a mistake to conclude that this result is statistically significant, saying this is less than .05, since the adjusted alpha for each test is now .01.

Multiple independent *t*-tests with Bonferroni adjustment tell us which pairs of the groups differ, but this does not capture the overall difference across groups since they only compare two groups per test. A better statistical test to identify group differences is **analysis of variance (ANOVA)**, which compares all groups simultaneously and so captures the overall differences across groups. ANOVA does not have to control for type I error as it conducts only one test. However, ANOVA only tells us that there exists a group difference; it does not tell us specifically which groups differ. Let us explain what we mean by this with an example in the next section.

Assumptions

All assumptions of an independent samples *t*-test still apply to one-way ANOVA, as it is a natural extension of an independent samples *t*-test. These parametric assumptions are as follows:

- The sampling distribution should be normal (i.e., the dependent variable should be normally distributed).
- The data should be measured at least on an interval level (i.e., continuous measurement).
- Variances in the groups in the comparison should be about the same.
- The measurements should be independent (i.e., subjects in the groups should not overlap).

Refer again to Chapter 8 for the details about how to check these assumptions.

Doing and Interpreting One-Way ANOVA

First, we need to set up hypotheses.

H_0: There is no significant difference among group means.

H_a: At least two group means differ.

or

$$H_0: \mu_1 = \mu_2 = \mu_3$$
$$H_a: \mu_j \neq \mu_k \text{ for } some \text{ } j \text{ and } k$$

and choose the level of significance from among .10, .05, .01, and .001. Again, the alternative hypothesis cannot be written as

$$H_a: \mu_j \neq \mu_k \text{ for } all \text{ } j \text{ and } k$$

because we do not know if all groups differ or if just two or three groups differ. The test statistic for one-way analysis of variance can be found by the following equation:

$$F = \frac{\text{Differences between groups}}{\text{Differences within groups}}$$

where both differences are shown in **Figure 11-9**. The associated *p*-value with this statistic is then compared with alpha, and the decision is made (i.e., the null hypothesis is rejected when the *p*-value associated with the computed statistic is smaller than the alpha or not rejected when the *p*-value associated with the computed statistic is larger than the alpha). From the statistic, it is clear that the differences between groups will be more likely to be statistically significant as the difference between groups gets larger (i.e., the statistic will likely fall in the rejection region as it gets larger).

The within-groups difference can be thought of as individual differences and is the variability in the data not explained by variables in the study (i.e., error). The between-groups difference can be easily shown

Figure 11-9

Visual representation of between- and within-group differences.

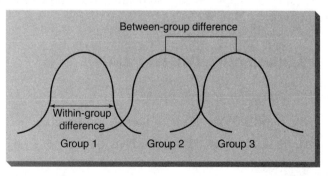

Figure 11-10

Undesirable effect of within-group differences in ANOVA.

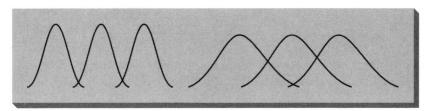

in the data in terms of means; this is the variability in the data that is explained by the variables in the study. When the variability explained by the variables under study is larger than that not explained by the variables under study, the results indicate that there is a statistically significant difference among groups. Note that a large within-group difference is not desirable, since it is more difficult to find the between-group difference when the individuals within groups are very dissimilar. In other words, the results may come out to be not significant even with substantial difference between means if individuals within groups differ greatly. Refer to **Figure 11-10** for an understanding of how the groups differ in the scenario on the left (less within-group difference) from the one on the right (more within-group difference).

To conduct a one-way ANOVA in SPSS, you can go to either Analyze > Compare means > One-way ANOVA or Analyze > Generalized linear models > Univariate as shown in **Figure 11-11** and **Figure 11-12**, respectively. The data shown in the figures represent the amount of exercise as an independent variable and health index as a dependent variable. We will first examine how to conduct one-way ANOVA in Analyze > Compare means > One-way ANOVA. In the One-Way ANOVA dialogue box, you will move an independent variable into "Factor" and a dependent variable into "Dependent List" by clicking the corresponding arrow buttons in the middle (see **Figure 11-13**). There are three buttons in the box; click on the "Options" button for now and check "Descriptives" and "Homogeneity of variance." Clicking "OK" will then produce the output of requested ANOVA analysis. Example output is shown in **Table 11-4**.

You will see that the health problem index for the no exercise group is 1.65, which seems to be lower than those of the other three groups. The group that exercised once a week showed a health index of 4.11,

Figure 11-11

Selecting one-way ANOVA under "Compare means" in SPSS.

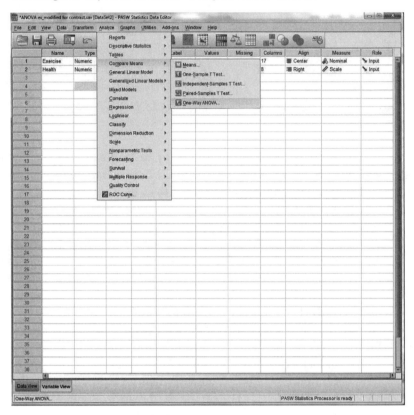

the group that exercised 3 days per week had a health index of 4.60, and the group that exercised 5 days per week showed a health index of 4.99. So, is the difference among these four groups statistically significant?

Levene's test results for the homogeneity of variance assumption indicate that this assumption is violated. This test again assumes the variances across the groups be equal, so a smaller p-value than α of 0.05, as shown in Table 11-4, leads us to reject the null hypothesis concluding that the variances are not the same. One thing to note here is that the sample sizes across all groups are the same. If so, one-way ANOVA is known to be robust to the violation of this assumption as well as that of normality. Therefore, we can somewhat ignore this violation.

Figure 11-12

Selecting one-way ANOVA under "Generalized linear models" in SPSS.

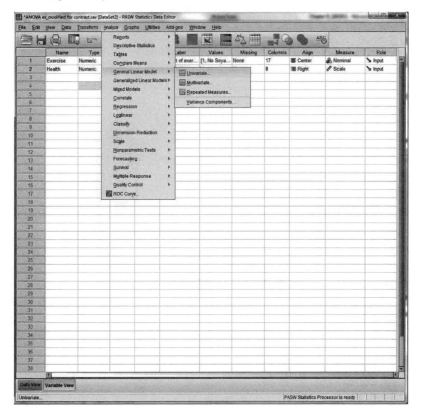

The ANOVA table shows the **F-statistic** (this is the statistical test reflecting the *F* distribution used in all ANOVAs) and the associated *p*-values of 2.636 and .056, respectively. Since the *p*-value is larger than our alpha of .05, the null hypothesis is not rejected, and it is determined that health index is not significantly different based on the amount of hours people exercise.

Reporting One-Way ANOVA

When reporting one-way ANOVA results, you should report the size of the *F*-statistic along with the associated degrees of freedom and associated

Figure 11-13

Defining variables in one-way ANOVA in SPSS.

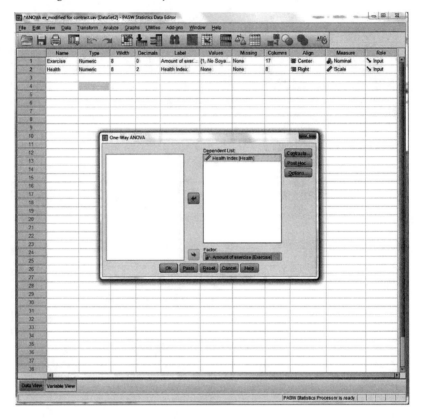

p-value. The effect size for one-way ANOVA results is called **omega squared** (ω^2) and is found with the following equation:

$$\omega^2 = \frac{\text{SSR} - df\text{R} \times \text{MSE}}{\text{SST} + \text{MSE}}$$

where SSR is the sums of squares for regression, dfR is the degrees of freedom for regression, MSE is the mean squares for residual, and SST is the total sums of squares. Note that ω^2 can only be calculated when the group sample sizes are equal.

The following is a sample report of our example.

- There was no significant effect of the amount of exercise per week on health index, $F(3, 76) = 2.64$, $p = .056$, $\omega = .24$.

Table	
11-4	Example Output of One-Way ANOVA in SPSS

Descriptives

Health Index

	N	Mean	Std. Deviation	Std. Error	95% Confidence Interval for Mean		Minimum	Maximum
					Lower Bound	Upper Bound		
None	20	4.9868	5.08437	1.13690	2.6072	7.3663	.35	21.08
1 day per week	20	4.6052	4.67263	1.04483	2.4184	6.7921	.33	18.47
3 days per week	20	4.1101	4.40991	.98609	2.0462	6.1740	.40	18.21
5 days per week	20	1.6530	1.10865	.24790	1.1341	2.1719	.31	4.11
Total	80	3.8388	4.26048	.47634	2.8906	4.7869	.31	21.08

ANOVA

Health Index

	Sum of Squares	df	Mean Square	F	Sig.
Between groups	135.130	3	45.043	2.636	.056
Within groups	1298.853	76	17.090		
Total	1433.983	79			

MULTIPLE COMPARISONS

In our previous example, no further analysis is needed since the amount of exercise did not make a significant difference on the health index. But what if there was a significant difference? As discussed, the significant result from a one-way ANOVA only tells us that at least two groups differ. Therefore, we need to conduct further analyses to find out which groups specifically differ from the other groups; these analyses are called planned contrasts and post hoc tests.

Doing and Interpreting Multiple Comparisons

Orthogonal planned contrasts, sometimes called a priori tests, are used when specific comparisons are determined *prior to* an examination of the data because you expect specific means to differ. These comparisons are oftentimes theory driven and protect us from overly increasing type I error. To set orthogonal planned contrasts, there are some rules to follow when choosing the theory-driven comparisons:

- Rule #1: Groups that are included in the comparison get either positive or negative weights. Groups that have positive weights are compared with groups that have negative weights.
- Rule #2: Groups that are excluded from the comparison get zero weights.
- Rule #3: The sum of all weights in the comparison adds up to zero.

Let us assume that we found the effect of the amount of exercise significantly differed in our previous example and we are specifically interested in whether exercising more than 3 days a week improves the health index. We then apply positive weights of +1 to 3 days per week and 5 days per week and negative weights of −1 to none and 1 day per week. These weights create orthogonal planned contrasts, as they sum up to zero.

Consider next that we are interested in whether exercising even 1 day per week improves the health index. We then apply a positive weight of +3 to none and negative weights of −1 to 1 day per week, 3 days per week, and 5 days per week. These weights sum up to zero, so they are orthogonal planned contrasts. These example contrast weights are summarized in **Table 11-5**.

To conduct planned contrasts in SPSS, you click on the "Contrasts" button in the One-Way ANOVA dialogue box, as shown in **Figure 11-14**;

Table					
11-5	**Example Contrast Weights**				

	None	1 Day per Week	3 Days per Week	5 Days per Week
Example 1	−1	−1	+1	+1
Example 2	+3	−1	−1	−1

Figure 11-14

Selecting "Contrasts" in the One-Way ANOVA dialogue box in SPSS.

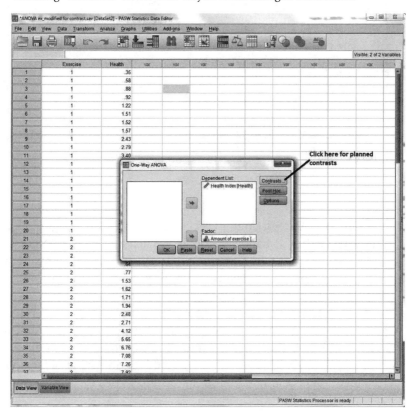

Figure 11-15

The One-Way ANOVA Contrasts dialogue box in SPSS.

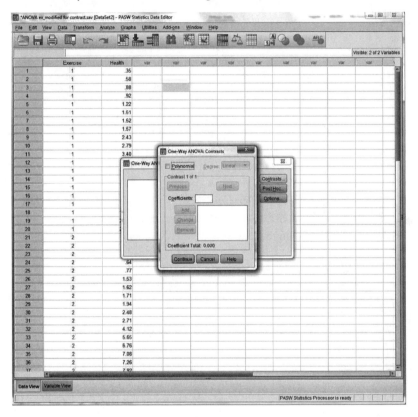

the One-Way ANOVA Contrasts dialogue box is shown in **Figure 11-15**. The exercise data set has been modified so that the one-way ANOVA results become significant, and it is used to explain multiple comparisons. You type the proposed coefficients in the One-Way ANOVA Contrasts dialogue box, in order, from the first group. For example, we would enter $-1, -1, +1$, and $+1$ in order for our first example and $+3, -1, -1$ and -1 for the second example. Note that you need to click on "Add" for each coefficient. Then, click "Continue" and proceed as you did with one-way ANOVA. This procedure will produce the output of requested planned contrasts. An example output is shown in **Table 11-6**.

Contrast Coefficients

Contrast		Amount of Exercise			
	No Soya Meals	1 Day per Week	3 Days per Week	5 Days per Week	
1	−1	−1	1	1	

Contrast Tests

		Contrast	Value of Contrast	Std. Error	t	df	Sig. (2-tailed)
Health index	Assume equal variances	1	−4.5459	2.02545	−2.244	76	.028
	Does not assume equal variances	1	−4.5459	2.025459	−2.244	54.767	.029

Post hoc tests are used when you want to make comparisons *after* examining the data to determine which means are contributing the greatest amount of variance by comparing all possible pairs of means. Note that comparing all possible pairs of means increases as the number of groups increases. For example, there are three tests of mean pairs when there are three groups (i.e., 1 vs. 2, 1 vs. 3, and 2 vs. 3). However, this number increases to six when there are four groups to compare pairwise (i.e., 1 vs. 2, 1 vs. 3, 1 vs. 4, 2 vs. 3, 2 vs. 4, and 3 vs.4). Post hoc tests control for inflated type I error. There are many post hoc tests available; however, we will only discuss the ones that are most commonly used. As shown in **Figure 11-17**, the post hoc tests are divided into two groups: ones that assume homogeneity of variance and the others that do not assume homogeneity of variance.

The first group is composed of tests that assume homogeneity of variance; most post hoc tests fall into this group. The most commonly used tests are the Bonferroni test, the Tukey test, and the Scheffe test. All of these tests take some steps to control type I error so that it would not be inflated by conducting many comparisons. Either the Bonferroni test or the Tukey test is good when the number of comparisons is low, but the Tukey test is better when the number of comparisons is high (i.e., the number of comparisons is more than five).

The second group is composed of tests that do not assume homogeneity of variance, so they are useful when this assumption is violated. There are four different tests, but Dunnett's C test is most commonly used for correcting the problem associated with type I error.

To conduct post hoc tests in SPSS, you click on the "Post Hoc" button in the One-Way ANOVA dialogue box as shown in **Figure 11-16**. The post hoc dialogue box is seen in **Figure 11-17**; note that the two groups of post hoc tests are shown. Select one of the post hoc tests in the dialogue box, depending on whether or not you violate the assumption of homogeneity of variance, and then click "Continue" to proceed as you did with one-way ANOVA. This procedure will produce the output of requested post hoc tests. An example output is shown in **Table 11-7**.

Reporting Planned Contrasts and/or Post Hoc Tests

When reporting planned contrast results, you can report as you would with independent samples *t*-test results. The following is a sample

Figure 11-16

Selecting "Post Hoc" in the One-Way ANOVA dialogue box in SPSS.

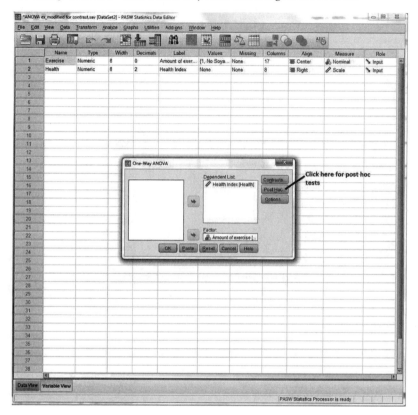

report of our first planned contrast, where we compare groups that exercise 3 days or more per week against those who exercise fewer than 3 days.

- Planned contrasts indicated that exercising 3 days or more per week significantly decreases the number of health problems than exercising fewer than 3 days per week, $t(76) = -2.24$, $p = .028$, $r = .06$.

When reporting post hoc test results, the p-value of each comparison along with the corresponding group descriptive statistics should

Figure 11-17

The Post Hoc dialogue box in SPSS.

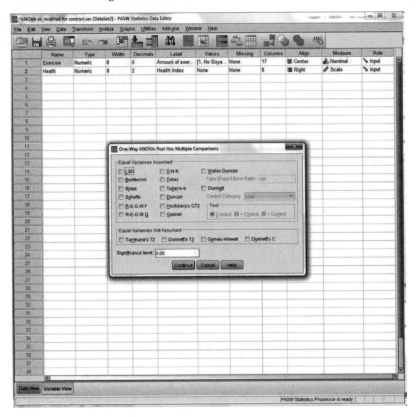

be reported, such as in this example reporting of a Bonferroni post hoc test:

- A Bonferroni post hoc test indicates that there was a significant difference on the health index between the group who do not exercise and the group who exercised 5 days per week, $p < .05$. The group who did not exercise had a higher problem index ($M = 5.49$, $SD = 6.03$) than the group who exercised 5 days per week ($M = 1.60$, $SD = 1.05$).

One-way ANOVA with planned contrasts combined with post hoc tests is a very robust approach to testing hypotheses on a single dependent variable.

Table	
11-7	Example Output of Post Hoc Tests

Multiple Comparisons
Health Index
Bonferroni

(I) Amount of Exercise	(J) Amount of Exercise	Mean Difference (I − J)	Std. Error	Sig.	95% Confidence Interval Lower Bound	95% Confidence Interval Upper Bound
None	1 day per week	.71412	1.43221	1.000	−3.1658	4.5941
	3 days per week	1.37655	1.43221	1.000	−2.5034	5.2565
	5 days per week	3.88351*	1.43221	.050	.0036	7.7635
1 day per week	None	−.71412	1.43221	1.000	−4.5941	3.1658
	3 days per week	.66242	1.43221	1.000	−3.2175	4.5424
	5 days per week	3.16939	1.43221	.179	−.7106	7.0493
3 days per week	None	−1.37655	1.43221	1.000	−5.2565	2.5034
	1 day per week	−.66242	1.43221	1.000	−4.5424	3.2175
	5 days per week	2.50696	1.43221	.504	−1.3730	6.3869
5 days per week	None	−3.88351*	1.43221	.050	−7.7635	−.0036
	1 day per week	−3.16939	1.43221	.179	−7.0493	.7106
	3 days per week	−2.50696	1.43221	.504	−6.3869	1.3730

* The mean difference is significant at the 0.05 level.

SUMMARY

In this chapter, we have seen how to conduct statistical tests that make comparisons between means. ~~The simplest statistic for comparing two means is the *t*-test.~~ The *t*-test and its variations allow us to make comparisons between two groups on a single dependent variable that is measured at the interval or ratio level. When we need to ~~make comparisons between more than two groups~~ and conserve power, ~~we turn to analysis of variance~~. One-way ANOVA allows us to make comparisons between three or more groups on a single dependent variable.

All these techniques share similar assumptions related to normality, independence, and homogeneity of variance. Tests of differences between means are most useful in descriptive comparative and experimental designs in which differences between groups are of interest.

Critical Thinking Questions

1. What statistical test would be most appropriate to examine differences between a sample mean and a population mean? Differences between men and women on exercise frequency? Differences between four ethnic groups on caloric intake?
2. What does "homogeneity of variance" mean in relation to conducting a one-way ANOVA?
3. How is the independent sample *t*-test different from the dependent sample difference test?
4. What multiple comparison tests would be most helpful following analysis of covariance?
5. How does the number of groups influence the choice of a statistical test of difference?
6. How would you report the following one-way ANOVA findings in APA style where an independent variable was nurses' education level?

ANOVA Patient Satisfaction					
	Sum of Squares	df	Mean Square	F	Sig.
Between groups	16.785	1	16.785	2.539	.114
Within groups	647.965	98	6.612		
Total	664.750	99			

7. How might you use the findings from the above ANOVA table in practice?

Self-Quiz www

1. Suppose you plan to compare systolic blood pressure among three age groups: 50–65, 66–80, and 80 and older. What statistical test will be most appropriate?
   a. One-way ANOVA
   b. One-sample *t*-test
   c. Independent *t*-test
   d. Dependent *t*-test
2. You are planning to test the effect of music therapy on chronic pain intensity among a single group of older adults in long-term care. What statistical test will be appropriate to determine if a significant difference on pain intensity is present before and after treatment in a single group?
   a. One-way ANOVA
   b. One-sample *t*-test
   c. Independent *t*-test
   d. Dependent *t*-test
3. You find that there is a significant mean difference among three different ethnicity groups on risk for falls in a nursing

home and want to find out which group differs specifically from which group. What procedure will help you determine such differences?

a. Bonferroni test

b. Levine's test for homogeneity

c. Post hoc or planned contrast

REFERENCE

Saban, K. L., Smith, B. M., Collins, E. G., & Bender Pape, T. L. (2011). Sex differences in perceived life satisfaction and functional status one year after severe traumatic brain injury. *Journal of Women's Health, 20*(2), 179–186. doi: 10.1089=jwh.2010.2334

Chapter

12

Tests for Comparing Group Means: Part II

Learning Objectives

The principal goal of this chapter is to explain the purpose of advanced statistical tests of differences between means (difference tests), when they may be used, and how to interpret the results. Because these advanced techniques require specialized skills to carry out, we would expect researchers and clinicans to consult with a statistician when using these approaches. This chapter will prepare you to:

- Understand the approaches to difference testing to answer complex research questions
- Evaluate assumptions of advanced difference tests
- Distinguish how the number of groups influences the choice of statistical test of difference
- Distinguish one-way analysis of variance (ANOVA) from more advanced ANOVA designs, such as factorial ANOVA, repeated measure ANOVA, ANCOVA, and multivariate ANOVA
- Correctly report the findings in APA style
- Understand how advanced tests of differences are used in evidence-based practice

Key Terms

Analysis of covariance (ANCOVA)

Assumption of sphericity

Box's M test

Covariates

Factorial analysis of variance

Multivariate

Multivariate analysis of
   covariance (MANCOVA)

Multivariate analysis of
   variance (MANOVA)

Simple effect analysis

Sphericity-assumed statistics

Univariate

INTRODUCTION

We have discussed tests of mean difference such as *t*-tests and analyses of variance (ANOVA) when there is one categorical independent variable and one continuous dependent variable. However, in practice you are likely to be interested in analyzing more than one independent and/or dependent variable, or you may be called upon to interpret findings from studies in which there is more than one independent or dependent variable. For example, it is likely that starting smoking is associated with several factors, such as exposure to smoking in a family environment, access to tobacco products, and cognitive capacity, which means there are three independent variables: exposure, access, and cognition. Similarly, we may believe that interventions to help people quit smoking must also help them maintain their current weight—so there are two dependent variables, smoking cessation and weight. We can also be interested in effects over multiple time points or multiple dependent and independent variables.

In these cases, you may run separate ANOVAs for each combination of variables, but you again run into the problem of inflated type I error that we have discussed in the previous chapter. Better alternatives are more advanced ANOVA designs that allow you to test multiple hypotheses simultaneously and test for interaction effects among multiple independent variables, if any. These tests require that dependent variables be continuous or measured at the interval or ratio level, while independent variable(s) must be categorical. In this chapter, we will discuss a number of advanced statistical tests that compare group means of continuous variable(s).

Case Study

Hawkins, S. Y. (2010). Improving glycemic control in older adults using a videophone motivational diabetes self-management intervention. *Research and Theory for Nursing Practice: An International Journal, 24*(4), 217–232.

You may recall from Chapter 2 we discussed an interesting study conducted by Shelley Y. Hawkins (2010), titled "Improving Glycemic Control in Older Adults Using a Videophone Motivational Diabetes Self-Management Intervention" and published in *Research and Theory for Nursing Practice: An International Journal*. Dr. Hawkins writes that the study was designed to test the effect of a videophone motivational interviewing (MI) diabetes self-management education (DSME) intervention on glycemic control among rural older adults. In this experimental study, Hawkins hypothesized that the effect of the intervention would continue over time and that the intervention and level of self-efficacy would influence glycemic control. Hawkins used a repeated-measures ANOVA to test the first hypothesis—effect of the intervention over time—and a factorial ANOVA to test the interaction effect of the intervention and self-efficacy on glycemic control. Hawkins found a statistically significant difference between the experimental group mean values and the control group over time. Moreover, the combination of the intervention with high self-efficacy in contrast to low self-efficacy produced a statistically significant decrease in HbA1c ($p = .043$).

Hawkins's study is a good example of the use of advanced ANOVA techniques. Nurses are often interested in complex human behaviors and other phenomena that cannot be explained or predicted by a single variable. Advanced ANOVAs make it possible to examine the complexity using a powerful test.

CHOOSING THE RIGHT STATISTICAL TEST

Choosing the right statistical test depends upon the proposed research questions and consideration of factors such as the number of independent and/or dependent variables. When group differences on the mean are examined for a single continuous (measured at the interval or ratio level) dependent variable, the design is called **univarate**, and tests like analysis of covariance, repeated measures analysis of variance, and **factorial analysis of variance** can be used. However, when there are two or more continuous dependent variables, the design is called multivariate and tests such as multivariate analysis of variance should be used to answer the proposed research question. It is not difficult to differentiate between univariate and multivariate tests since the number of dependent variables is usually reported in an article or clearly stated in a hypothesis. However, we recommend that you pay special attention to the discussion of independence in Chapter 11, because whether the groups are independent or dependent is often times confusing.

Another important consideration is the number of independent variables. Elsewhere, we worked on examples where there was only one independent variable. However, we are often interested in research that examines the effect of more than one independent variable on the dependent variable(s). For example, you may be interested in investigating the effect of ethnicity (measured in three groups of white, black, or Asian) as well as gender (male or female) on attitudes towards abortion. When there is more than one independent variable in group comparison tests, you now need to look at potential interaction effects between/among these independent variables as they may work together to create group differences. For example, male Asians may have more negative attitudes towards abortion than female whites or vice versa. Therefore, we recommend you that you pay special attention to our discussions on interaction effects in a later section.

ANALYSIS OF COVARIANCE (ANCOVA)

In a previous section, we saw how one-way ANOVA allowed us to examine group differences on a continuous dependent variable. However, in many studies there may be another continuous variable that may affect the dependent variable, but is not a variable of interest. These variables are known as **covariates** and can be included in ANOVA to control for their unwanted effect on the dependent variable. Let us assume that we are still interested in examining the effect of the amount of exercise on a health problem index, but we know that weight will also affect the health problem index score. We can get a better understanding of the influence of weight if we measure the weight and enter it as a covariate in an ANOVA design. Such a procedure will allow us to control for the effect of weight and discern the true effect of the amount of exercise on the health problem index.

When we identify covariates that truly affect the dependent variable and carefully control for them in an **analysis of covariance (AN-COVA)**, we achieve an important goal; we can explain the variability that we could not explain without the covariates. The unexplained variability is reduced, and the design allows us to examine more accurately the true effect of an independent variable. The partitioning of the variability is shown in **Figure 12-1**.

Assumptions

ANCOVA has all of the assumptions of ANOVA, plus an additional two assumptions. These are: (1) independence between the covariate and independent variable and (2) homogeneity of regression slope.

Figure 12-1

Partitioning of variability in analysis of covariance (ANCOVA).

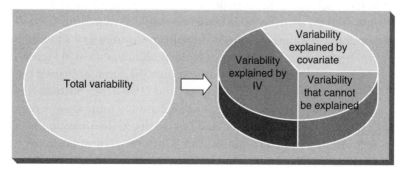

Independence between the covariate and independent variable make sense as we try to reduce the variability that is not explained by the independent variable by explaining it with the covariates. If they are not independent, the variability that is explained will be difficult to interpret and it will not be clear whether it was explained by an independent variable.

Homogeneity of regression slope means that the relationship between the covariate and the dependent variable stays the same. For example, the health problem index should increase as the weight increases in the various workout groups if the health problem index also increases as the weight increases in the group who does not exercise at all.

Doing and Interpreting ANCOVA

First, we need to set up hypotheses. These look similar to those of ANOVA design, except the means are adjusted for the covariate:

H_0: There is no significant difference among group means.

H_a: At least two group means differ.

or

$$H_0: \mu_1 = \mu_2 = \mu_3$$
$$H_a: \mu_j \neq \mu_k \text{ for some } j \text{ and } k$$

Select the level of significance from among .10, .05, .01 and .001.

To conduct ANCOVA in SPSS, go to Analyze > Generalized linear models > Univariate as shown in **Figure 12-2**. The data here are those we used in the multiple comparison example where the amount of exercise significantly affected the health problem index. In the Univariate dialogue box, you will move an independent variable, Exercise, into "Fixed Factor(s)," a dependent variable, Health, into "Dependent Variable," and the covariate, Weight, into "Covariate(s)" by clicking the corresponding "arrow" buttons in the middle as shown in **Figure 12-3**. There are six buttons in the box, but only the commonly used buttons are discussed here. The "Contrasts" and "Post Hoc" buttons are used when further investigations are needed among more than two groups in the factor with significant ANOVA results, as discussed in the earlier section on planned contrasts. The "Options" button gives us several choices that may help us interpret the results of factorial ANOVA, and

Figure 12-2

Selecting ANCOVA under "Generalized Linear Models" in SPSS.

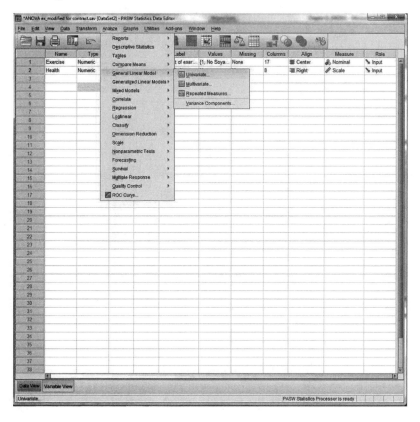

these are shown in **Figure** 12-4. Please review the example output shown in **Table 12-1**.

You will see that the ANCOVA results table looks very similar to that of a one-way ANOVA, but there is an additional line representing the covariate, weight. The result indicates that weight significantly affects the health problem index, as the *p*-value is less than .05. However, you will find it interesting that the amount of exercise does not have a significant effect on the health problem index with the covariate in the design. Remember that the amount of exercise had a significant effect on health problem index in one-way ANOVA? When we add the covariate, weight, to our analysis, we find that weight is significantly

Figure 12-3

Defining variables in ANCOVA in SPSS.

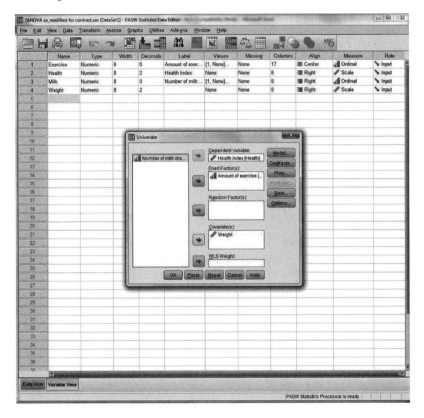

affecting the health problem index, cancelling out the effect of exercise. If we had neglected to include the covariate of weight, we would have misinterpreted the influence of exercise on the health problem index.

Reporting ANCOVA

When reporting ANCOVA results, you should report the size of the F-statistics along with associated degrees of freedom and associated p-value. For an effect size for ANCOVA, omega squared (ω^2) can be calculated as it is with one-way ANOVA. ω^2 is only useful when the sample sizes for all groups are the same. Another type of effect size,

Figure 12-4

Useful options for ANCOVA in SPSS.

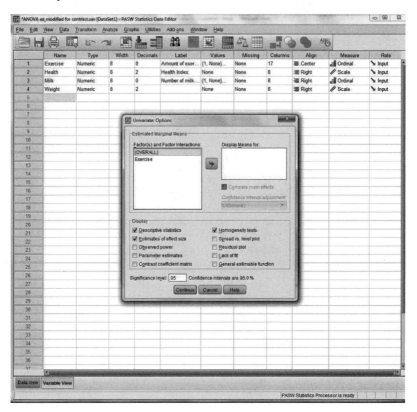

partial eta squared (η^2), is useful when sample sizes are not equal, and this can be obtained in SPSS.

The following is a sample report from our example:

- The covariate, weight, was significantly affecting this sample's health problem index, $F(1, 75) = 11.53$, $p = .001$, $\eta^2 = .13$. However, the amount of exercise per week did not significantly affect the health problem index after controlling for the effect of weight, $F(3, 75) = 1.79$, $p = .156$, $\eta^2 = .07$.

Further group comparisons of the amount of exercise per week are not considered, as the overall test was not significant.

Table	
12-1	Example Output of ANCOVA in SPSS

Between-Subjects Factors

		Value Label	N
Amount of exercise	1	None	20
	2	1 day per week	20
	3	3 days per week	20
	4	5 days per week	20

Tests of Between-Subjects Effects
Dependent Variable: Health Index

Source	Type III Sum of Squares	df	Mean Square	F	Sig.
Corrected model	378.918[a]	4	94.730	5.258	.001
Intercept	54.409	1	54.409	3.020	.086
Weight	207.643	1	207.643	11.525	.001
Exercise	96.883	3	32.294	1.792	.156
Total	3005.774	80			
Corrected total	1730.203	79			

[a] R squared = .219 (adjusted R squared = .177)

FACTORIAL ANALYSIS OF VARIANCE (ANOVA)

One-way ANOVA allows us to examine the effect of one independent grouping variable on a dependent variable, which is why the design is called *one-way* ANOVA. However, it is oftentimes the case that a researcher wants to examine the effect of more than one independent grouping variable on a dependent variable. For example, we may be interested in examining the effect of both the amount of exercise and the number of servings of soy milk drunk per day on the health problem index. In this case, factorial ANOVA is used to examine the joint effect of the two independent variables, and the design is called *two-way* factorial ANOVA because there are two independent variables. You can see that with large sample sizes, there is the potential for three-, four-, and five-way (etc.) factorial ANOVA, but this text will only consider two-way factorial ANOVA. In factorial ANOVA, each level of each factor (independent variable) is crossed with each level of another factor so that we can examine the interaction effect between factors. In our present example, we would examine the mean differences between one serving of soy milk per day and no exercise per week, one serving of soy milk and one day of exercise per week, one serving of soy milk and three days of exercise per week, then two servings of soy milk and one day of exercise per week, etc. (you get the idea). (See **Table 12-2**.) An interaction effect is said to be present when the differences explained by one factor are dependent upon those by the other factor.

Doing and Interpreting Factorial ANOVA

First, we need to set up hypotheses. Since we have two independent factors, we need hypotheses for each of the factors and another for the interaction effects between the two factors.

> H_{01}: There is no significant difference among group means in Factor A.
>
> H_{a1}: At least two group means in Factor A differ.

or

$H_{01}: \mu_1 = \mu_2 = \mu_3$

$H_{a1}: \mu_j \neq \mu_k$ for some j and k

> H_{02}: There is no significant difference among group means in Factor B.
>
> H_{a2}: At least two group means in Factor B differ.

> H_{03}: There is no significant interaction effect between Factor A and B.
>
> H_{a3}: There is a significant interaction effect between Factor A and B.

Then, we need to select the level of significance from among .10, .05, .01, and .001.

Table 12-2	Example Permutations of a Two-Way Factorial ANOVA			
		Factor A (Amount of Exercise)		
	None (A1)	1 Day per Week (A2)	3 Days per Week (A3)	5 Days per Week (A4)
Factor B (servings of soy milk) None (B1)	A1B1	A2B1	A3B1	A4B1
1 cup of milk (B2)	A1B2	A2B2	A3B2	A4B2
2 cups of milk (B3)	A1B3	A2B3	A3B3	A4B3
3 cups of milk (B4)	A1B4	A2B4	A3B4	A4B4

The test statistic for each hypothesis in factorial analysis of variance can be found by the same equation:

$$F = \frac{\text{Differences between groups}}{\text{Differences within groups}}$$

where differences between groups are divided into three components: (1) differences between groups explained by Factor A, (2) differences between groups explained by Factor B, and (3) differences between groups explained by the interaction of Factors A and B. The associated p-value with this statistic is then compared with alpha and the decision is made (i.e., the null hypothesis is rejected when the p-value associated with the computed statistic is smaller than the alpha or not rejected when the p-value associated with the computed statistic is larger than the alpha).

Results are reported as main effect and interaction effect. The main effect is the group difference between of each of the independent (grouping) variables on the dependent variables. The interaction effect reflects the interaction of grouping variables on the dependent variables. Be sure to look at the interaction effect first, as you must be careful in interpreting the main effect when the interaction effect is significant—that is, the results of main effect cannot be trusted when the effect of one factor is associated with the effect of another factor. In that case, you need to conduct a **simple effect analysis**, which looks at the effect of one variable at each level of the other variable to see if the results of a given main effect happen at all levels of the other variable. On the other hand, the main effect results can be interpreted, as they are when the interaction effect is not significant.

To conduct a two-way factorial ANOVA in SPSS, go to Analyze > General Linear Model > Univariate, as shown in **Figure 12-5**. The variables shown in Figure 12-6 represent the amount of exercise and the number of servings of soy milk consumed per day as independent variables, and health problem index as a dependent variable. In the Univariate dialogue box, you will move independent variables into "Fixed Factor(s)" and a dependent variable into "Dependent Variable" by clicking corresponding arrow buttons in the middle as shown in **Figure 12-6**. There are six buttons in the box, but only the commonly used buttons are discussed here. The "Contrasts" and "Post Hoc" buttons are used when further investigations are needed among more than two groups in the factor with significant ANOVA results as discussed

Figure 12-5

Selecting factorial ANOVA under "General Linear Model" in SPSS.

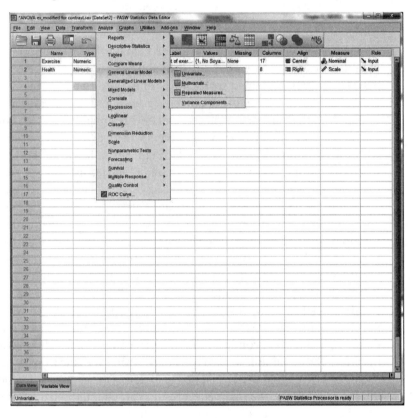

in the earlier section on planned contrasts. The "Plots" button can be used to help us interpret the interaction effect visually and can be created as shown in **Figure 12-7**. The "Options" button gives us several choices that may help us interpret the results of factorial ANOVA; these are shown in **Figure 12-8**. Clicking "OK" will then produce the output of the requested factorial ANOVA analysis. Example output is shown in **Table 12-3**.

You will see that the Levene's test for the assumption of homogeneity of variance is violated, but ANOVA designs tend to be robust when the sample sizes across the groups are the same. From the interaction

Figure 12-6

Defining variables in factorial ANOVA in SPSS.

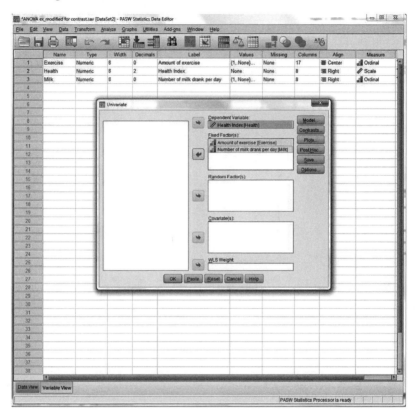

plot (Profile Plots), we can see that the lines look relatively parallel to each other. When the lines in the interaction plot are parallel, we say that there is no interaction effect between the two factors; if not, there is an interaction effect. In this case, there is no interaction between servings of soy milk per day and level of exercise.

In the "Test of Between-Subjects Effects" table, the two main factors (exercise and amount of milk consumed) were found to have significant effects on the health index, but the interaction between them was not significant. Since one factor is not dependent upon the other factor from its nonsignificant results (i.e., one factor does not work with the other

Figure 12-7

Creating an interaction plot in factorial ANOVA in SPSS.

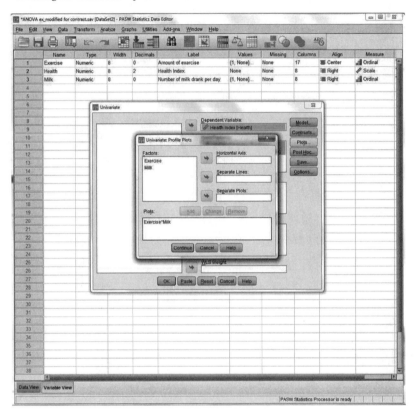

factor to make changes on means of the dependent variable), the main effects can be interpreted as they are. Both the amount of exercise and the amount of milk consumed per day have a significant effect on the health problem index, but we still do not know how the groups (levels of exercise or amount of milk consumed) differ. Therefore, Bonferroni tests on both factors should be done as post hoc tests; these results are shown in **Table 12-4**. From the outputs, we can see that people who exercise 0 or 1 day per week have significantly more health problems than people who exercise 5 days per week. We can also see that people who drank 3 cups of soy milk have significantly fewer health problems than those who drank less than 3 cups of soy milk.

Figure 12-8

Useful options for factorial ANOVA in SPSS.

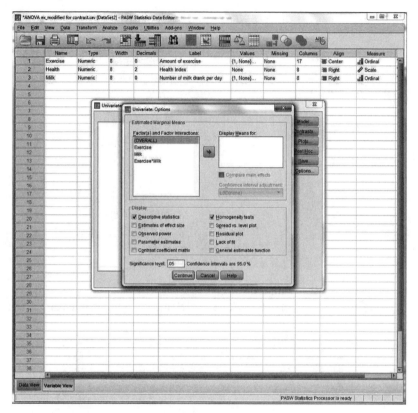

Reporting Two-Way Factorial ANOVA

Reporting two-way factorial ANOVA results is similar to that in one-way ANOVA. You should report the size of *F*-statistics along with associated degrees of freedom and associated *p*-value for both the main effects and interaction effect. The computation of effect size for any factorial ANOVA design is more complicated and cumbersome than that for one-way ANOVA; therefore, the numeric derivation is omitted in this text.

Table	
12-3	Example Output of Factorial ANOVA in SPSS

Between-Subjects Factors

		Value Label	N
Amount of exercise	1	None	20
	2	1 day per week	20
	3	3 days per week	20
	4	5 days per week	20
Amount of milk drunk per day	1	None	20
	2	1 cup of milk	20
	3	2 cups of milk	20
	4	3 cups of milk	20

Descriptive Statistics
Dependent Variable: Health Index

Amount of Exercise	Amount of Milk Drunk . . .	Mean	Std. Deviation	N
None	None	2.9376	4.02726	3
	1 cup of milk	1.9706	1.74597	4
	2 cups of milk	5.9369	6.62055	8
	3 cups of milk	9.1084	7.21533	5
	Total	5.4866	6.03848	20
1 day per week	None	1.3453	1.03013	4
	1 cup of milk	2.1023	2.34922	6
	2 cups of milk	4.0644	2.46577	5
	3 cups of milk	11.4266	5.16764	5
	Total	4.7725	5.00301	20
3 days per week	None	2.4256	1.87489	8
	1 cup of milk	2.1997	1.10954	6
	2 cups of milk	2.2205	1.22501	2
	3 cups of milk	11.2894	5.14213	4
	Total	4.1101	4.40991	20

(continued)

Amount of Exercise	Amount of Milk Drunk . . .	Mean	Std. Deviation	N
5 days per week	None	1.2470	.93219	5
	1 cup of milk	1.1051	.32208	4
	2 cups of milk	1.4355	1.24393	5
	3 cups of milk	2.3715	1.07419	6
	Total	1.6031	1.05270	20
Total	None	1.9917	1.95122	20
	1 cup of milk	1.9057	1.56504	20
	2 cups of milk	3.9718	4.63435	20
	3 cups of milk	8.1031	6.06176	20
	Total	3.9931	4.67988	80

Levene's Test of Equality of Error Variances[a]
Dependent Variable: Health Index

F	df1	df2	Sig.
3.496	15	64	.000

Tests the null hypothesis that the error variance of the dependent variable is equal across groups.
a. Design: Intercept + Exercise + Milk + Exercise × Milk

Tests of Between-Subjects Effects
Dependent Variable: Health Index

Source	Type III Sum of Squares	df	Mean Square	F	Sig.
Corrected model	884.306[a]	15	58.954	4.460	.000
Intercept	1114.192	1	1114.192	84.299	.000
Exercise	149.809	3	49.936	3.778	.015
Milk	571.097	3	190.366	14.403	.000
Exercise × milk	181.024	9	20.114	1.522	.159
Error	845.898	64	13.217		
Total	3005.774	80			
Corrected total	1730.203	79			

a. R squared = .511 (adjusted R squared = .397)

(continued)

Table	
12-3	Continued

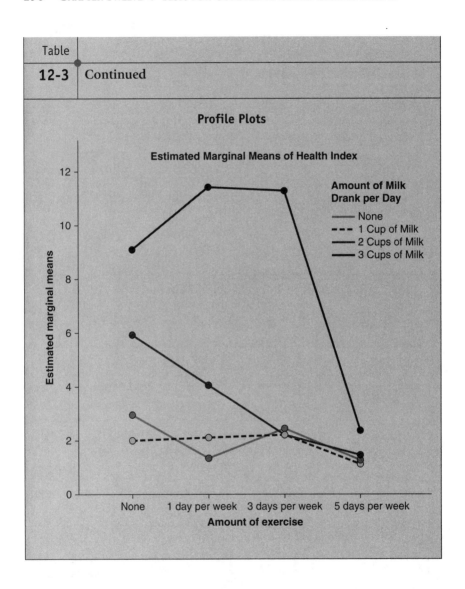

Table	
12-4	**Post Hoc Test Results of Factorial ANOVA in SPSS**

Amount of Exercise

Multiple Comparisons
Health Index
Bonferroni

(I) Amount of Exercise	(J) Amount of Exercise	Mean Difference (I − J)	Std. Error	Sig.	95% Confidence Interval	
					Lower Bound	Upper Bound
None	1 day per week	.7141	1.14966	1.000	−2.4161	3.8443
	3 days per week	1.3765	1.14966	1.000	−1.7537	4.5068
	5 days per week	3.8835*	1.14966	.007	.7533	7.0137
1 day per week	None	−.7141	1.14966	1.000	−3.8443	2.4161
	3 days per week	.6624	1.14966	1.000	−2.4678	3.7926
	5 days per week	3.1694	1.14966	.046	.0392	6.2996
3 days per week	None	−1.3765	1.14966	1.000	−4.5068	1.7537
	1 day per week	−.6624	1.14966	1.000	−3.7926	2.4678
	5 days per week	2.5070	1.14966	.197	−.6233	5.6372
5 days per week	None	−3.8835*	1.14966	.007	−7.0137	−.7533
	1 day per week	−3.1694*	1.14966	.046	−6.2996	−.0392
	3 days per week	−2.5070	1.14966	.197	−5.6372	.6233

Based on observed means.
The error term is mean square (error) = 13.217.
* The mean difference is significant at the .05 level.

(continued)

Table	
12-4	Continued

Amount of Milk Drunk per Day

Multiple Comparisons
Health Index
Bonferroni

(I) Amount of Milk Drunk per Day	(J) Amount of Milk Drunk per Day	Mean Difference (I − J)	Std. Error	Sig.	95% Confidence Interval Lower Bound	Upper Bound
None	1 cup of milk	.0859	1.14966	1.000	−3.0443	3.2162
	2 cups of milk	−1.9801	1.14966	.539	−5.1103	1.1501
	3 cups of milk	−6.1114*	1.14966	.000	−9.2417	−2.9812
1 cup of milk	None	−.0859	1.14966	1.000	−3.2162	3.0443
	2 cups of milk	−2.0661	1.14966	.462	−5.1963	1.0642
	3 cups of milk	−6.1974*	1.14966	.000	−9.3276	−3.0672
2 cups of milk	None	1.9801	1.14966	.539	−1.1501	5.1103
	1 cup of milk	2.0661	1.14966	.462	−1.0642	5.1963
	3 cups of milk	−4.1313*	1.14966	.004	−7.2616	−1.0011
3 cups of milk	None	6.1114*	1.14966	.000	2.9812	9.2417
	1 cup of milk	6.1974*	1.14966	.000	3.0672	9.3276
	2 cups of milk	4.1313*	1.14966	.004	1.0011	7.2616

Based on observed means.
The error term is mean square (error) = 13.217.
* The mean difference is significant at the .05 level.

The following is a sample report of our example:

- There was no significant interaction effect between the amount of exercise per week and the number of servings of soy milk drunk per day on the health problem index, $F(9, 64) = 1.52$, $p = .159$.
- There was a significant effect of the amount of exercise per week on the health index, $F(3, 64) = 3.78$, $p = .015$. The Bonferroni test revealed that the group who exercised 5 days per week had a

significantly lower health problem index than both groups who did not exercise and who exercised 1 day per week (both $p < .05$).
- There was also a significant effect of the number of servings of soy milk drunk per day on health index, $F(3, 64) = 14.40$, $p = .000$. The Bonferroni test revealed that the group who drank three cups of soy milk per day had significantly lower health problem index than any other group (all $p < .01$).

REPEATED MEASURES ANALYSIS OF VARIANCE (ANOVA)

Introduction

Until now, we have discussed ANOVA designs where several independent group means are compared. However, there are situations where several group means come from the same group of participants, similar to what we discussed in dependent samples *t*-test. Repeated measures ANOVA is simply an extended design of dependent samples *t*-test where there are more than two repeated measurements in the same group of participants. Recall that repeated measures design can take two different forms. The first is when the same variable is measured multiple times on the same group of participants to see changes, and the second is when multiple treatments are given to the same group of participants to compare responses to each treatment. Repeated measures ANOVA can also be used when sample members are matched based on some important characteristic. For example, male and female nursing home residents may be matched when a researcher is interested in examining the level of sleep disturbance, since they reside in the same environment.

Repeated measures ANOVA design provides the following advantages:

- It is suitable when some variables are to be measured repeatedly over time (i.e., longitudinal design).
- It is an economical design compared to independent sample group comparison since the sample size is smaller than when you have more than one group.
- Since it analyzes only one group, the variability is lower than in multigroup design and therefore the validity of results will be higher.

However, there are disadvantages:

- Repeated measurements may not be possible due to dropout, death, etc.
- There may be a maturation effect where the subjects change over the course of the study.
- There may be other effects that reduce the validity of results, such as subjects' scores heading toward to the average with multiple measurements.

Assumptions

Repeated measures ANOVA assumptions are very similar to those required by one-way ANOVA, such as normality and homogeneity of variance. Just like other ANOVA designs, repeated measures ANOVA is robust to the violation of the normality and homogeneity of variance, especially when group sample sizes are the same. Note that the assumption of homogeneity of variance only applies when there are groups that are compared along with repeated measures. However, the last assumption of independence is automatically violated because the measurements are coming from the same group of participants. Instead, the assumption of relations between/among repeated measures is added. The last assumption is called the **assumption of sphericity**, which means that the variances of the differences as well as the correlations among the repeated measures are all equal.

Doing and Interpreting Repeated Measures ANOVA

First, we need to set up hypotheses.

H_0: There is no significant difference among repeated measure means.

H_1: At least two repeated measure means differ.

or

$$H_{01}: \mu_1 = \mu_2 = \mu_3$$
$$H_{a1}: \mu_j \neq \mu_k \text{ for some } j \text{ and } k$$

Choose the level of significance from among .10, .05, .01, and .001.

Figure 12-9

Selecting repeated measures ANOVA under "General Linear Model" in SPSS.

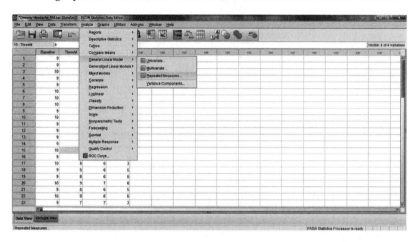

The test statistic for each hypothesis in repeated measures ANOVA can be found by the same equation:

$$F = \frac{\text{Differences between time measurements}}{\text{Differences within each measurement}}$$

The associated *p*-value with this statistic is then compared with alpha and the decision is made (i.e., the null hypothesis is rejected when the *p*-value associated with the computed statistic is smaller than the alpha or not rejected when the *p*-value associated with the computed statistic is larger than the alpha).

To conduct a repeated measures ANOVA in SPSS, you go to Analyze > General linear model > Repeated measures, as shown in **Figure 12-9**. This will bring up the Repeated Measures Define Factor(s) dialogue box; here, the name of the within-subject factor and the number of repeated measures should be identified as shown in **Figure 12-10**. In this example, the data is the number of falls across four times: baseline, 3 months after, 6 months after, and 9 months after implementing a newly developed fall prevention intervention. Type "Fall" for name and "4" for level since there are four measurements, then click "Define." In the Repeated Measures dialogue box, you will see that four levels with questions marks are already shown under "Within-Subjects

Figure 12-10

Defining the name and level of repeated measures in repeated measures ANOVA in SPSS.

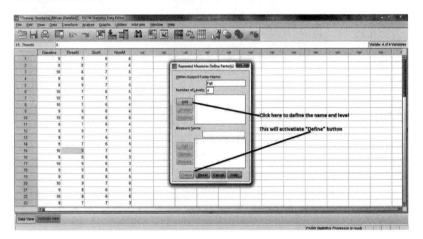

Variable(s)," so now you need to tell SPSS what those levels are. Move corresponding levels starting with the first measurement, in this case "baseline," until every level is moved by clicking an arrow button in the middle as shown in **Figure 12-11**. There are six buttons in the box, but only the commonly used buttons are discussed here. The

Figure 12-11

Defining variables in repeated measures ANOVA in SPSS.

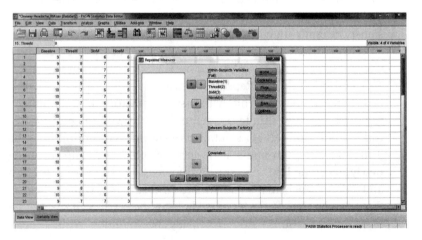

Figure 12-12

Useful options for repeated measures ANOVA in SPSS.

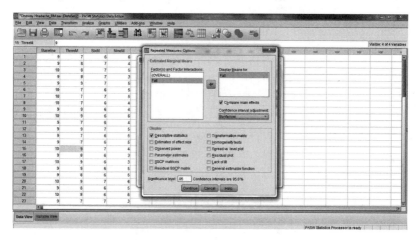

"Contrasts" and "Post Hoc" buttons are used when further investigations are needed among more than two groups in the factor with significant ANOVA results, as discussed earlier. Again, the overall significance test in repeated measures ANOVA only tells that there is a significant difference between time measurements. It does not tell which measurements differ from the other measurements. The "Options" button provides several options that may help us interpret the results of repeated measures ANOVA, and these are shown in **Figure 12-12**. Clicking "OK" will then produce the output of the requested analysis. Example output is shown in **Table 12-5**.

You will see that the group sample sizes are the same (in the Descriptive Statistics section) with no missing data (as seen in Table 12-5) and the assumption of sphericity is violated with a *p*-value of less than .05. If this assumption was not violated, **sphericity-assumed statistics** could be interpreted and reported from the "Tests of Within-Subjects Effects" section of the table as you would for one-way ANOVA. However, this result will be biased when the assumption of sphericity is violated. Although this may sound scary, the "Tests of Within-Subjects Effects" section also generates other statistics that adjust for this violation, and one of these can be reported instead. There are different recommendations with regard to which one to use, but it is often

Table	
12-5	**Example Output of Repeated Measures ANOVA in SPSS**

Within-Subjects Factors
Measure: MEASURE_1

Fall	Dependent Variable
1	Baseline
2	ThreeM
3	SixM
4	NineM

Descriptive Statistics

	Mean	Std. Deviation	N
Baseline	9.42	.499	50
ThreeM	7.96	.880	50
SixM	6.54	.503	50
NineM	4.70	1.035	50

Multivariate Tests[b]

Effect		Value	F	Hypothesis df	Error df	Sig.
Fall	Pillai's trace	.960	378.556[a]	3.000	47.000	.000
	Wilks' lambda	.040	378.556[a]	3.000	47.000	.000
	Hotelling's trace	24.163	378.556[a]	3.000	47.000	.000
	Roy's largest root	24.163	378.556[a]	3.000	47.000	.000

[a] Exact statistic

[b] Design: intercept

Within subjects design: fall

(continued)

Mauchly's Test of Sphericity[b]							
					Epsilon[a]		
Within-Subjects Effect	Mauchly's W	Approx. Chi-Square	df	Sig.	Greenhouse–Geisser	Huynh–Feldt	Lower Bound
Fall	.646	20.837	5	.001	.776	.817	.333

Tests the null hypothesis that the error covariance matrix of the orthonormalized transformed dependent variables is proportional to an identity matrix.

[a] May be used to adjust the degrees of freedom for the averaged tests of significance. Corrected tests are displayed in the Tests of Within-Subjects Effects section.

[b] Design: intercept

Within subjects design: fall

Tests of Within-Subjects Effects
Measure: MEASURE_1

Source		Type III Sum of Squares	df	Mean Square	F	Sig.
Fall	Sphericity assumed	609.175	3	203.058	350.862	.000
	Greenhouse–Geisser	609.175	2.329	261.578	350.862	.000
	Huynh–Feldt	609.175	2.452	248.430	350.862	.000
	Lower bound	609.175	1.000	609.175	350.862	.000
Error (fall)	Sphericity assumed	85.075	147	.579		
	Greenhouse–Geisser	85.075	114.113	.746		
	Huynh–Feldt	85.075	120.153	.708		
	Lower bound	85.075	49.000	1.736		

suggested to use Greenhouse–Geisser statistics when the estimates of epsilon in the Mauchly's test table is less than 0.75 and to use Huynh–Feldt statistics when it is larger than 0.75. In our example, epsilon is larger than 0.75, so Huynh–Feldt statistics should be used. Therefore, these repeated measures significantly differ, and each time measurement does significantly differ from each other from Bonferroni pairwise comparisons as shown in **Table 12-6.**

Table							
12-6	**Bonferroni Pairwise Comparisons**						

Pairwise Comparisons
Measure: MEASURE_1

(I) Fall	(J) Fall	Mean Difference (I − J)	Std. Error	Sig.[a]	95% Confidence Interval for Difference[a] Lower Bound	95% Confidence Interval for Difference[a] Upper Bound
1	2	1.460[*]	.128	.000	1.107	1.813
	3	2.880[*]	.106	.000	2.590	3.170
	4	4.720[*]	.164	.000	4.268	5.172
2	1	−1.460[*]	.128	.000	−1.813	−1.107
	3	1.420[*]	.140	.000	1.034	1.806
	4	3.260[*]	.195	.000	2.723	3.797
3	1	−2.880[*]	.106	.000	−3.170	−2.590
	2	−1.420[*]	.140	.000	−1.806	−1.034
	4	1.840[*]	.163	.000	1.393	2.287
4	1	−4.720[*]	.164	.000	−5.172	−4.268
	2	−3.260[*]	.195	.000	−3.797	−2.723
	3	−1.840[*]	.163	.000	−2.287	−1.393

Based on estimated marginal means.

* The mean difference is significant at the .05 level.

[a] Adjustment for multiple comparisons: Bonferroni

Reporting Repeated Measures Factorial ANOVA

Reporting repeated measures ANOVA results is similar to that in one-way ANOVA, but the result of Mauchly's test for sphericity should begin the reporting since it will determine which statistics to report. You should then report the size of F-statistics along with associated degrees of freedom and the associated p-value. The computation of effect size for any repeated measures ANOVA design is fairly complicated and more cumbersome than that for one-way ANOVA; therefore, the numeric derivation is omitted in this text.

The following is a sample report of our example.

- Mauchly's test indicated that the assumption of sphericity has been violated, χ^2 (5) = 20.84, p = .001; therefore, the Huynh–Feldt correction was used (ε = .82). The results show that the number of falls significantly changed over time, F (2.45, 120.15) = 350.86, p = .000. The Bonferroni post hoc test revealed that the number of falls was significantly lower in 9 months after fall prevention program than those in 6 months after, 3 months after, and baseline (all ps < .001). The number of falls in 6 months after fall prevention program was significantly lower than those in 3 months after, and baseline, and the number of falls in 3 months after was also significantly lower than that of baseline (all ps < .001).

MULTIVARIATE ANALYSIS OF VARIANCE (MANOVA)

Introduction

Multivariate analysis of variance (MANOVA) is simply an extension of ANOVA where group differences on more than one dependent variable are investigated. For example, we might be interested in studying the effect of exercise frequency on weight and bone density. We could group participants into low-, moderate-, and high-exercise-frequency groups, then examine that effect on the two dependent variables: weight and bone density. You may think of conducting multiple one-way ANOVAs, but like multiple t-tests the type I error will be inflated and you will not be able to capture information about the relationship among those dependent variables. MANOVA has the power to detect significant group differences along a combination of dependent variables, and so it is a better design than several one-way ANOVAs in this situation.

Multivariate procedures are very useful when you have multiple dependent variables to investigate simultaneously. However, you should keep in mind that the design would be much more complicated because there is more than one dependent variable. You may want to limit the number of dependent variables based on the manageability and alignment with the theory guiding the research. Too many dependent variables will confuse the results and make it difficult to convey the meaning of the study.

Assumptions

All of the ANOVA assumptions are also required for MANOVA, but in a multivariate way. Multivariate normality is assumed in MANOVA, but there is no way of checking this assumption in SPSS. Therefore, you should check if each dependent variable is normally distributed as in ANOVA. Independence assumption can be easily checked, but homogeneity of variance in MANOVA means something a little different and needs another approach. Since there is more than one dependent variable, there are covariances between dependent variables as well as variance in each dependent variable. Levene's test will only be able to test for equality of variability, but there is a multivariate statistic that can test for equality of variance–covariance, named **Box's M test**. The theory is the same as Levene's test, in that it assumes the equality of variance–covariance among the variables and the assumption is said to be violated when the test result is significant. As with ANOVA, MANOVA is also relatively robust to the violation of assumptions when the sample sizes across groups are the same.

Doing and Interpreting MANOVA

First, we need to set up hypotheses. The data contains nurses' education level as an independent variable and the number of patient falls, functional ability, and quality of life as dependent variables. Since we have three dependent variables, we need hypotheses for each variable.

H_0: There is no significant difference between group means on any of the dependent variables.

H_a: There is a significant difference between group means on some of the dependent variables.

Choose the level of significance from among .10, .05, .01, and .001.

The test statistic for each hypothesis in repeated measures MANOVA can be found by the same equation:

$$F = \frac{\text{Differences between groups}}{\text{Differences within groups}}$$

The associated *p*-value with this statistic is then compared with alpha and the decision is made (i.e., the null hypothesis is rejected when the *p*-value associated with the computed statistic is smaller than the alpha or not rejected when the *p*-value associated with the computed statistic is larger than the alpha).

If the results of MANOVA come out to be significant, it tells us that the groups differ on the combination of dependent variables, but it does not specify on which dependent variable(s) the groups differ. There are several ways of following up the significant results from MANOVA, including:

- One-way ANOVA: Significant results of MANOVA can be followed by a series of one-way ANOVAs for each dependent variable, with Bonferroni adjustment for type I error, to see on which dependent variable the groups differ.
- Discriminant analysis: This procedure is the exact opposite of MANOVA. It uses dependent variables in MANOVA as predictor variables and the groups as the dependent variable. Its goal is to predict group membership with predictor variables, and it allows assessing the relative importance of each dependent variable in predicting group membership.
- Roy–Bargman stepdown analysis: This procedure assesses the importance of each dependent variable using the most important dependent variable as a covariate in steps.

Since both discriminant analysis and Roy–Bargman stepdown analysis are advanced techniques beyond the scope of this text, only a series of one-way ANOVAs with Bonferroni adjustment for type I error will be discussed as a follow-up test of MANOVA in this text.

To conduct MANOVA in SPSS, go to Analyze > General linear model > Multivariate, as shown in **Figure 12-13**. In the Multivariate dialogue box, move independent variables into "Fixed Factor(s)" and dependent variables into "Dependent Variables" by clicking the corresponding arrow buttons in the middle (see **Figure 12-14**). Notice the space for dependent variables is wider than that found in univariate

Figure 12-13

Selecting MANOVA under "General Linear Model" in SPSS.

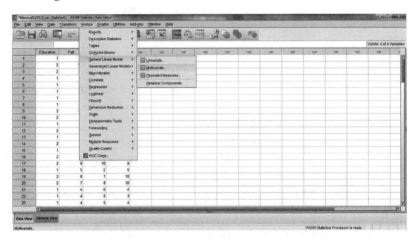

general linear models. There are six buttons in the box, but only commonly used buttons are discussed here. The "Contrasts" and "Post Hoc" buttons are used when further investigations are needed among more than two groups in the factor with significant ANOVA results as discussed in an earlier section. However, we do not have to use these

Figure 12-14

Defining variables in MANOVA in SPSS.

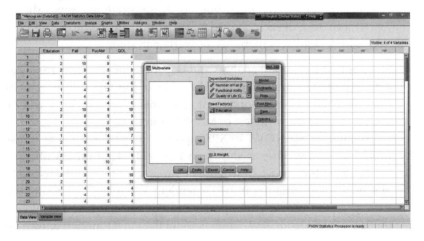

Figure 12-15

Useful options for MANOVA in SPSS.

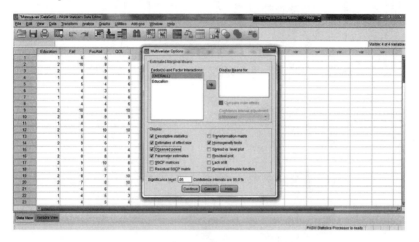

buttons since we have only two groups. The "Options" button provides several options that may help us interpret the results of factorial ANOVA; these are shown in **Figure 12-15**. Clicking "OK" will then produce the output of the requested MANOVA analysis. Example output is shown in **Table 12-7**.

The output indicates that the independent variable, nurses' education level, has a significant effect on the combined dependent variables of number of falls, functional ability, and quality of life with a significant p-value of .000. Note that the output reports four different statistics for the effect of the independent variable, including Pillai's trace, Wilks' lambda, Hotelling's trace, and Roy's largest root. These statistics will report the same results in most situations with relatively good robustness to the violation of multivariate normality like in our output, but there may be some cases where not all statistics agree on the significance of the independent variable(s). If dissimilarity among statistics happens, the decision can be made based on which set of dependent variables group differences occurs, but refer to previous research for the further discussion (Olson, 1974, 1976; Stevens, 1980). Separate univariate ANOVAs performed as a follow-up test indicated that nurses' education level had a significant effect on all dependent variables.

Table
12-7 | Example Output of MANOVA in SPSS

Multivariate Tests^c

Effect		Value	F	Hypothesis df	Error df	Sig.	Partial Eta Squared	Noncent. Parameter	Observed Power^b
Intercept	Pillai's trace	.978	1454.679^a	3.000	96.000	.000	.978	4364.036	1.000
	Wilks' lambda	.022	1454.679^a	3.000	96.000	.000	.978	4364.036	1.000
	Hotelling's trace	45.459	1454.679^a	3.000	96.000	.000	.978	4364.036	1.000
	Roy's largest root	45.459	1454.679^a	3.000	96.000	.000	.978	4364.036	1.000
Education	Pillai's trace	.621	52.336^a	3.000	96.000	.000	.621	157.009	1.000
	Wilks' lambda	.379	52.336^a	3.000	96.000	.000	.621	157.009	1.000
	Hotelling's trace	1.636	52.336^a	3.000	96.000	.000	.621	157.009	1.000
	Roy's largest root	1.636	52.336^a	3.000	96.000	.000	.621	157.009	1.000

[a] Exact statistic   [b] Computer using alpha = .05   [c] Design: intercept + education

ANOVA

		Sum of Squares	df	Mean Square	F	Sig.
Number of falls	Between groups	200.255	1	200.255	68.203	.000
	Within groups	287.745	98	2.936		
	Total	488.00	99			
Functional ability	Between groups	117.749	1	117.749	49.154	.000
	Within groups	234.761	98	2.396		
	Total	352.510	99			
Quality of life	Between groups	140.701	1	140.701	54.600	.000
	Within groups	252.539	98	2.577		
	Total	393.240	99			

Reporting MANOVA

Reporting MANOVA results is little bit different from that in one-way ANOVA because it uses different statistics. You should include one of the four multivariate statistics that are reported in the output along with the size of F-statistics, associated degrees of freedom, and the associated p-value. The follow-up ANOVAs' results are reported as shown previously.

The following is a sample report of our example:

- There was a significant effect of nurses' education level on the combined dependent variables of number of falls, functional ability, and quality of life, $\Lambda = 0.38$, $F(3, 96) = 52.34$, $p = .000$. Separate univariate ANOVAs were followed up; the overall significance revealed that nurses' education level had a significant effect on all of the dependent variables: number of falls, $F(1, 98) = 68.20$, $p = .000$, functional ability, $F(1, 98) = 49.15$, $p = .000$, and quality of life, $F(1, 98) = 54.60$, $p = .000$.

Note that this reporting uses Wilks' lambda, but you could choose the others. You will have to ensure that you use the corresponding symbol to report (i.e., V for Pillai's trace, T for Hotelling's trace, and Θ for Roy's largest root).

Nurse researchers and clinicans occasionally encounter studies and analyses that include an extension of MANOVA, **multivariate analysis of covariance (MANCOVA)** and factorial MANOVA. While this discussion is beyond the scope of our text, you should understand that MANCOVA is used to to control for the effect of covariates on the combination of dependent variables and factorial MANOVA is used to investigate both main and interaction effect of independent variables on a combination of dependent variables.

SUMMARY

In this chapter, we have seen how to conduct advanced statistical tests to make comparisons between means. Occasionally, it will be important to control other variables that we think may influence the dependent variable, and we can accomplish this by employing analysis of covariance (ANCOVA). Other variations of ANOVA include factorial and repeated measures, which are specialized applications of one-way ANOVA that are applicable in situations when there are multiple independent variables or the same variable is being measured over time. Multivariate analysis of variance (MANOVA) allows us to analyze the effects of the grouping variable(s) on more than one dependent variable.

All these techniques share similar assumptions related to normality, independence, and homogeneity of variance. Once we are examining multiple independent or dependent variables, we also need to conduct statistical tests that tell us more specifically which variables are creating the effect.

Tests of differences between means are most useful in descriptive comparative and experimental designs in which differences between groups are of interest.

Critical Thinking Questions

1. What are the differences between one-way analysis of variance (ANOVA) and factorial ANOVA, repeated measures ANOVA, ANCOVA, and multivariate ANOVA?
2. Why is ANCOVA a more powerful design than one-way ANOVA when there is a third variable that is affecting a relationship between the independent and dependent variable?
3. How do statistically significant interaction effects influence the interpretation of main effects in factorial ANOVA?

Self-Quiz

1. Suppose you plan to compare systolic blood pressure between three age groups (50–65 years, 66–80, and 80 and older), and evidence from the literature suggests that weight may influence blood pressure. What statistical test will be most appropriate?
   a. One-way ANOVA
   b. Analysis of covariance
   c. Independent *t*-test
   d. MANOVA

2. Suppose you find that there is an interaction effect of gender and ethnicity on risk for falls in a nursing home. What statistic will help you determine which variable is contributing the greatest variance?
   a. Simple effect analysis
   b. Bonferroni test
   c. Levine's test for homogeneity
3. Suppose you find that there is a significant effect of the independent variable on the set of four dependent variables. Which test(s) can you conduct to follow up the significant results?
   a. A series of ANOVAs
   b. Roy–Bargman stepdown analysis
   c. Discriminant analysis
   d. All of the above

REFERENCES

Hawkins, S. Y. (2010). Improving glycemic control in older adults using a videophone motivational diabetes self-management intervention. *Research and Theory for Nursing Practice: An International Journal, 24*(4), 217–232.

Olson, C. L. (1974). Comparative robustness of six tests in multivariate analysis of variance. *Journal of the American Statistical Association, 69,* 894–908.

Olson, C. L. (1976). On choosing a test statistic in multivariate analysis of variance. *Psychological Bulletin, 83,* 579–586.

Stevens, J. P. (1980). Power of the multivariate analysis of variance tests. *Psychological Bulletin, 88,* 728–737.

Chapter

13

Nonparametric Tests

Learning Objectives

The principal goal of this chapter is to explain nonparametric tests as counterparts of parametric tests for group comparisons when the assumptions of parametric tests are violated. This chapter will prepare you to:

- Distinguish between parametric tests and nonparametric tests
- Evaluate assumptions of nonparametric tests of differences
- Distinguish between independent sample difference tests and dependent sample difference tests
- Distinguish between two samples and more than two samples difference tests
- Report the necessary findings correctly in APA style
- Understand the application of nonparametric tests in evidence-based practice

Key Terms

Group comparisons

Kruskal–Wallis test

Mann–Whitney test

Nonparametric

Parametric

Wilcoxon rank-sum test

Wilcoxon signed-rank test

WHY NONPARAMETRIC TESTS?

Up to this point, we have discussed different types of **parametric** tests, such as the independent *t*-test, and have stated that these tests have a certain set of assumptions that usually include a distributional assumption such as normality. For the best statistical results, we need to ensure that assumptions of normal distribution and others are met before the analysis. Sometimes the researcher or clinician decides to use a parametric test even when one or more violations of the assumptions are present. Parametric statistical tests can still be a good choice in such circumstances if the violations are not serious. However, there are occasions where serious violations of these assumptions occur. Of course, we may try to deal with the violation through transformations, but transformations do not always solve distributional problems and parametric tests cannot be used in such situations. We might ask if, under such circumstances, we should abandon our pursuit of the analysis? Thankfully, we have another set of options.

When data are not normally distributed, we can use **nonparametric tests (tests that do not rely on a probability distribution)** that are counterparts of parametric tests. Most nonparametric tests analyze the rank of the data, not the actual raw data. In general, parametric tests tend to be a little more powerful than nonparametric tests when the assumptions are met. However, nonparametric tests become more powerful in detecting significant results when distributional assumptions are violated.

Case Study

Kneipp, S. M., Kairalla, J. A., Lutz, B. L., Pereira, D., Hall, A. G., Flocks, J., . . . Schwartz, T. (2011). Public health nursing case management for women receiving Temporary Assistance for Needy Families: A randomized controlled trial using community-based participatory research. *American Journal of Public Health*, *101*(9), 1759–1768.

In 2011, Shawn M. Kneipp and colleagues published a study in the *American Journal of Public Health* on the effectiveness of a case management intervention to promote use of healthcare visits, Medicaid knowledge and skill, and health and functional status among women with chronic health conditions who were receiving Temporary Assistance for Needy Families (TANF). They employed an experimental design and randomly assigned 432 women to a public health nurse for case management plus Medicaid intervention or a control group. Medicaid outcomes were measured pre- and post-training.

This design would seem to lend itself very well to analysis of variance, but the researchers found that Medicaid knowledge and skills were not distributed normally in the population. They used the Wilcoxon matched-pairs signed ranks test instead and found that Medicaid knowledge and skills improved ($P < .001$ for both) as a result of the intervention.

Nonparametric tests serve the same purposes as their parametric counterparts but allow us to take a more conservative approach to analysis when some aspect of the test assumptions is being violated.

COMPARING TWO INDEPENDENT GROUPS: WILCOXON RANK-SUM TEST AND/OR MANN–WHITNEY TEST

When the distributional assumption of independent samples *t*-test is violated, the nonparametric counterparts should be used, and these are the **Wilcoxon rank-sum test** and the **Mann–Whitney test**. These tests are useful for making **group comparisons** when parametric assumptions cannot be met.

Let us consider an example where we compare family satisfaction with dementia care between a traditional caregiver group ($N = 13$) and a music therapy group ($N = 9$). We know that because these sample sizes are small, the distribution will not be normal; therefore, either the Wilcoxon rank-sum test or the Mann–Whitney test will be an appropriate test for this situation. The data are shown in **Table 13-1**.

Table 13-1	Data for Dementia Care Example	
Traditional Caregiver Group		**Music Therapy Group**
1		21
12		25
17		29
15		27
9		9
15		15
17		27
19		19
13		16
7		
16		
3		
14		

Assumptions

As these are nonparametric tests, there are no distributional assumptions. However, these tests do assume the following:

- Random samples
- Two groups are independent of each other
- Level of measurements is at least ordinal

Doing and Interpreting Wilcoxon Rank-Sum Test and/or Mann–Whitney Test

First, we need to set up hypotheses; these are the same as those of an independent samples t-test:

H_0: The distributional functions are identical for two groups.

H_a: The distributional functions are not identical for two groups.

Select the level of significance from among .10, .05, .01, and .001.

The test statistics for both tests are calculated using ranks of the data. When the group sample sizes are equal, the test statistics are the summed rank value that is smaller than the other. However, it will be the summed rank value of the group with the smaller sample size if the group sample sizes are not equal. For our example, the sum of rank value in the traditional caregiver group is 109.50, and that in the music therapy group is 143.50. Due to the unequal sample sizes, our test statistic is the summed rank value for the music therapy group.

Once the statistic is computed, the associated *p*-value is then compared with alpha and the decision is made (i.e., the null hypothesis is rejected when the *p*-value associated with the computed statistic is smaller than the alpha or not rejected when the *p*-value associated with the computed statistic is larger than the alpha).

To conduct Wilcoxon rank-sum tests and/or Mann–Whitney tests in SPSS, go to Analyze >Nonparametric tests > Legacy dialogs > 2 Independent Samples, as shown in **Figure 13-1**. In the Two Independent Samples Tests dialogue box, move a dependent variable, family satisfaction, ("Fam Sat") into "Test Variable List" and an independent variable, "Treatment," into "Grouping Variable" by clicking the corresponding arrow buttons in the middle (**Figure 13-2**). You will notice that "Mann–Whitney U" is checked by default under "Test Type"; this option will produce statistics of both Wilcoxon rank-sum tests and Mann–Whitney tests.

Figure 13-1

Selecting Mann–Whitney tests in SPSS.

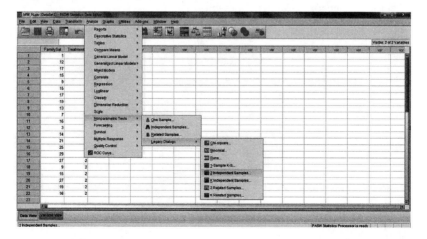

Figure 13-2

Defining variables in Mann–Whitney Tests in SPSS.

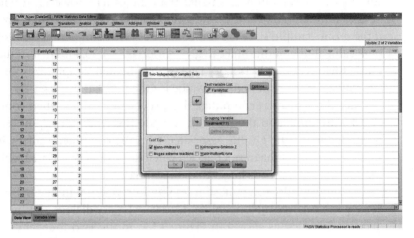

You will notice that the "OK" button is not active because we have not yet defined our two groups. As you see in **Figure 13-3**, we have defined the coding of 1 for the traditional caregiver group and 2 for the music therapy group. Now click on the "Define Groups" button and assign 1 for group 1 and 2 for group 2, as in **Figure 13-4**. Clicking "Continue" and then "OK" will produce the output. Example output is shown in **Table 13-2**. With

Figure 13-3

Coding scheme for "Treatment" variable.

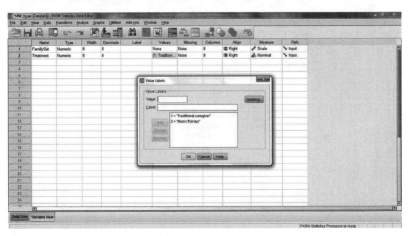

Figure 13-4

Defining groups in Mann–Whitney tests in SPSS.

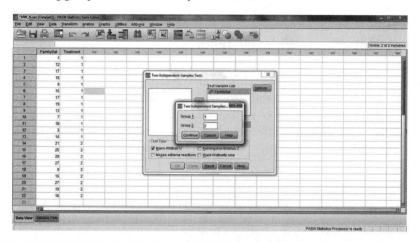

Table	
13-2	**Example Output of Mann–Whitney Tests in SPSS**

Ranks

Treatment		N	Mean Rank	Sum of Ranks
FamilySat	Traditional caregiver	13	8.42	109.50
	Music therapy	9	15.94	143.50
	Total	22		

Test Statistics[b]

	FamilySat
Mann–Whitney U	18.500
Wilcoxon W	109.500
Z	−2.678
Asymp. sig. (2-tailed)	.007
Exact sig. [2 × (1-tailed sig.)]	.006[a]

[a] Not corrected for ties.
[b] Grouping variable: treatment

a significant *p*-value of .007, we can see that family satisfaction differs significantly depending upon the type of treatment.

Reporting Mann–Whitney Tests

When reporting Mann–Whitney test results, you should report the size of the corresponding statistics and associated *p*-value, as well as report medians of groups so that the readers will know how the sample statistics are different. Effect size, *r*, can be computed and reported with the following equation:

$$r = \frac{Z}{\sqrt{N}}$$

where *Z* is one of the statistics that SPSS calculates for Mann–Whitney tests and *N* is the total number of observations. The following is an example of how to report the test results.

- For Mann–Whitney tests: Family satisfaction levels in traditional caregiver group (*Mdn* = 14.00) did differ significantly from music therapy group (*Mdn* = 21.00), *U* = 18.50, *z* = −2.68, *p* = .007, *r* = −.57.
- For Wilcoxon rank-sum tests: Family satisfaction levels in the traditional caregiver group (*Mdn* = 14.00) differed significantly from music therapy group (*Mdn* = 21.00), W_s = 109.50, *z* = −2.68, *p* = .007, *r* = −.57.

COMPARING TWO DEPENDENT GROUPS: WILCOXON SIGNED-RANK TEST

When the distributional assumption of dependent samples *t*-test is violated, the counterparts of dependent samples *t*-test should be used. This test is called the **Wilcoxon signed-rank test**. Let us consider a comparison between the amount of memory loss before (*N* = 12) and after (*N* = 12) music therapy. We know that these sample sizes are small and the distribution will not be normal; therefore, the Wilcoxon

Table	
13-3	**Data for Music Therapy Example**

Before	After
9	21
15	25
11	29
12	27
7	9
13	15
17	27
12	19
13	16
16	14
16	30
13	21

signed-rank test should be used instead of the dependent samples *t*-test. The data are shown in **Table 13-3**.

Assumptions

As the Wilcoxon signed-rank test is the nonparametric counterpart of the dependent samples *t*-test, *t* does not have distributional assumptions. However, this test does assume the following:

- The sample is a random sample of a respective population
- Variable measurement is continuous
- The level of measurement is at least interval

You may wonder why the level of measurement is required to be continuous and at least the interval level of measurement. This is because the Wilcoxon signed-rank test uses ranks of the difference between the measurements, not the raw measurements, just as the dependent sample *t*-tests analyzes the difference between the means, not the raw scores.

Doing and Interpreting Wilcoxon Signed-Rank Tests

First, we need to set up hypotheses; these are the same as for the independent samples t-test:

H_0: The median of the difference between measurements is equal to zero.

H_a: The median of the difference between measurements is not equal to zero.

and choose the level of significance from among .10, .05, .01, and .001.

The test statistic is calculated using ranks of the data, but the signs of the difference between measurements are assigned to the corresponding rank with Wilcoxon signed-rank tests. The statistic is simply the sum of positive ranks of the difference between measurements, but the value of z in the SPSS output can be reported instead.

Once the statistic is computed, the associated p-value is then compared with alpha and the decision is made (i.e., the null hypothesis is rejected when p-value associated with the computed statistic is smaller than the alpha or not rejected when the p-value associated with the computed statistic is larger than the alpha).

To conduct a Wilcoxon signed-rank sum test in SPSS, go to Analyze > Nonparametric tests > Legacy dialogs > 2 related samples as shown in **Figure 13-5**. In the Two Related samples Tests dialogue box, you will move variables to be paired into "Test Pairs" in order by clicking

Figure 13-5

Selecting Wilcoxon signed-rank tests in SPSS.

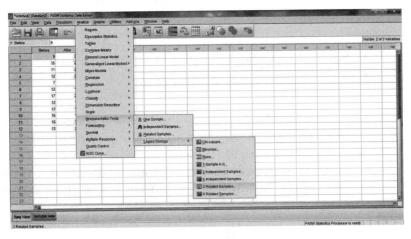

Figure 13-6

Defining variables in Wilcoxon signed-rank tests in SPSS.

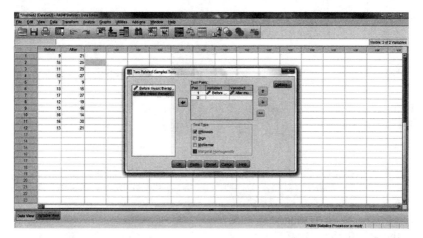

corresponding arrow buttons in the middle, as shown in **Figure 13-6**. You will notice that "Wilcoxon" is checked by default under "Test Type," and this option will produce statistics of Wilcoxon signed-rank tests. Notice that you can request descriptive statistics by clicking the "Options" button and then checking "Descriptives" in the Two Related Samples Options dialogue box (see **Figure 13-7**). Clicking "Continue"

Figure 13-7

Requesting descriptives for Wilcoxon signed-rank tests in SPSS.

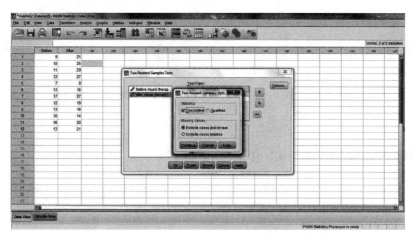

Table 13-4	Example Output of Wilcoxon Signed-Rank Tests in SPSS

Descriptive Statistics

	N	Mean	Std. Deviation	Minimum	Maximum
Before music therapy	12	12.83	2.949	7	17
After music therapy	12	21.08	6.680	9	30

Ranks

		N	Mean Rank	Sum of Ranks
After music therapy—before music therapy	Negative ranks	1[a]	2.00	2.00
	Positive ranks	11[b]	6.91	76.00
	Ties	0[c]		
	Total	12		

[a] After music therapy $<$ before music therapy
[b] After music therapy $>$ before music therapy
[c] After music therapy $=$ before music therapy

Test Statistics[b]

	After Music Therapy − Before Music Therapy
Z	−2.908[a]
Asymp. sig. (2-tailed)	.004

[a] Based on negative ranks   [b] Wilcoxon signed-ranks test

and then "OK" will then produce the output. Example output is shown in **Table 13-4**.

Reporting Wilcoxon Signed-Rank Tests

When reporting Wilcoxon signed-rank test results, you should report the size of corresponding statistics and associated *p*-value; also, be sure to report medians of repeated measurements so that the readers will know how the sample statistic is different. Effect size, *r*, can be computed and reported with the same equation as that of the Mann–Whitney test:

$$r = \frac{Z}{\sqrt{N}}$$

where *Z* is one of the statistics that SPSS calculates for Wilcoxon signed-rank tests and *N* is the total number of observations. The following is a sample report of our example:

- Family satisfaction levels were significantly greater after music therapy (*Mdn* = 21.00) than before music therapy (*Mdn* = 13.00), *z* = −2.91, *p* = .004, *r* = −.84.

COMPARING SEVERAL INDEPENDENT GROUPS: KRUSKAL–WALLIS TEST

One-way analysis of variance (ANOVA) is used when there are more than two group means to compare. The test is quite robust despite violation of the required assumptions as long as the sample sizes across groups are equal. However, there is a nonparametric counterpart that we can use when the assumptions are violated or when the sample size is too small; this is the **Kruskal–Wallis test**. Let us consider an example where we compare the effectiveness of dementia care among a traditional caregiver group (*N* = 13), a music therapy group (*N* = 9), and a medical treatment group (*N* = 10). We know that these sample sizes are small, so the distribution will not be normal; therefore, the Kruskal–Wallis test is appropriate instead of one-way ANOVA. The data are shown in **Table 13-5**.

Assumptions

Like the previously discussed nonparametric tests, Kruskal–Wallis tests do not have distributional assumptions. However, they assume the following:

- All samples are random samples from their respective populations.
- Three or more samples are independent of each other.
- Levels of measurements are at least ordinal.

Table 13-5	Data for Music Therapy Example	
Traditional Caregiver Group	**Music Therapy Group**	**Medical Therapy Group**
1	17	30
12	25	29
17	19	28
15	27	32
9	9	24
15	15	18
17	22	31
19	19	27
13	16	22
7		30
16		
3		
14		

Doing and Interpreting the Kruskal–Wallis Test

First, we need to set up hypotheses:

H_0: The distributional functions are identical for different groups.

H_a: The distributional functions are not identical for different groups.

and select the level of significance from among .10, .05, .01, and .001.

The test statistics for both tests are calculated using ranks of the data, and the numeric example of deriving the statistic is omitted in this text. Once the statistic is computed, the associated p-value is then compared with alpha and the decision is made (i.e., the null hypothesis is rejected when the p-value associated with the computed statistic is smaller than the alpha or not rejected when the p-value associated with the computed statistic is larger than the alpha). Like with one-way ANOVA, the significant results in Kruskal–Wallis tests only tell you that the groups differ. Further investigation can help parcel out the variance attributed by each; for this, the Mann–Whitney test can be used.

Figure 13-8

Selecting Kruskal–Wallis tests in SPSS.

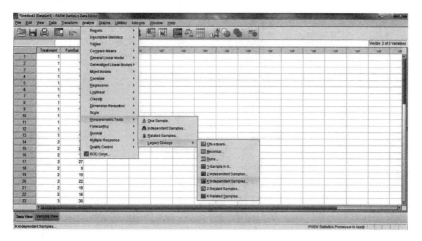

To conduct Kruskal–Wallis tests in SPSS, go to Analyze > Nonparametric tests > Legacy dialogs > K independent samples, as shown in **Figure 13-8**. In the Tests for Several Independent Samples dialogue box, you will move a dependent variable, "Family Satisfaction," into "Test Variable List" and an independent variable, "Treatment," into "Grouping Variable" by clicking the corresponding arrow buttons in the middle (**Figure 13-9**).

Figure 13-9

Defining variables in Kruskal–Wallis tests in SPSS.

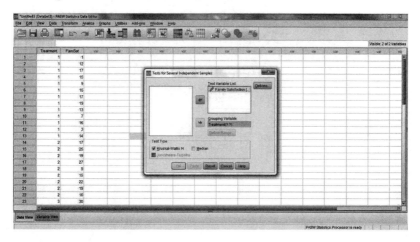

Figure 13-10

Range of a grouping variable.

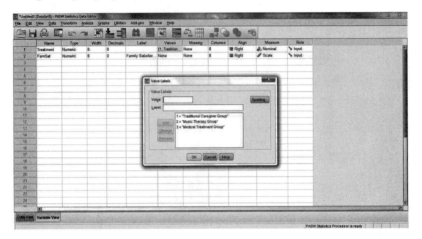

You will notice that "Kruskal–Wallis H" is checked by default under "Test Type"; this option will produce the statistic of the Kruskal–Wallis test. You will notice that the "OK" button is not still active; this is because we have not defined our groups. As you see in **Figure 13-10**, we have a total of three groups, so click on the "Define Groups" button and type in "1" for minimum and "3" for maximum (shown in **Figure 13-11**). Note that you

Figure 13-11

Defining groups in Kruskal–Wallis tests in SPSS.

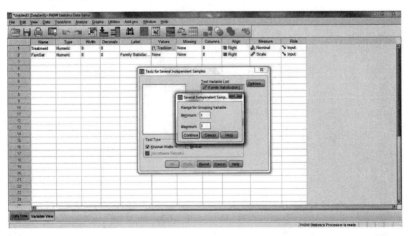

Table	
13-6	**Example Output of Kruskal–Wallis Tests in SPSS**

Ranks

	Treatment	N	Mean Rank
Family statisfaction	Traditional caregiver group	13	8.69
	Music therapy group	9	16.78
	Medical treatment group	10	26.40
	Total	32	

Test Statistics[a,b]

	Family Statisfaction
Chi-square	20.214
df	2
Asymp. sig.	.000

[a] Kruskal–Willis test
[b] Grouping variable: treatment

can request descriptive statistics if desired by clicking "Descriptives" under the "Option" button. Clicking "Continue" and then "OK" will produce the output. Example output is shown in **Table 13-6**. With a significant *p*-value of .000, we can see that family satisfaction differs significantly depending upon the type of treatment.

Reporting the Kruskal–Wallace Test

Reporting the Kruskal–Wallace test is very similar to other test results and should include the size of the corresponding statistics, associated *p*-value, and medians of groups.

The following is a sample report from the example.

- Family satisfaction level was significantly different depending on the type of treatment for dementia care, $H(2) = 20.21$, $p = .000$. Mann–Whitney tests with Bonferroni correction were used to follow up on the significant findings, and all effects are determined to be significant at .0167. The traditional caregiver group was different from both the musical therapy group ($U = 21.00$, $r = -.54$) and the medical treatment group ($U = 1.00$, $r = -.85$), and the musical therapy group was also different from the medical treatment group ($U = 10.00$, $r = -.61$).

COMPARING SEVERAL DEPENDENT GROUPS: FRIEDMAN'S ANOVA

Repeated-measures analysis of variance (ANOVA) is used when measurements are repeated more than two times, and Friedman's ANOVA is a nonparametric counterpart that can be used when the assumptions are violated or when the sample size is too small. For example, let us consider an example where we examine the change of memory loss among baseline ($N = 7$), 6 months after ($N = 7$), and 1 year after ($N = 7$) music therapy. We know that since these sample sizes are small, the distribution will not be normal; therefore, Friedman's ANOVA is the appropriate test. The data are shown in **Table 13-7.**

Table		
13-7	Friedman's ANOVA Data for Music Therapy Example	
Baseline	**3 Months After**	**6 Months After**
29	22	10
25	23	12
29	26	14
27	19	7
30	26	11
15	19	7
27	24	9

Assumptions

As Friedman's ANOVA is the nonparametric counterpart of repeated measures ANOVA, it does not have distributional assumptions. However, the following assumptions apply:

- Measurements are independent of each other.
- Levels of measurements are at least ordinal.

Doing and Interpreting Friedman's ANOVA

First, we need to set up hypotheses, and they are the same as those of repeated measures ANOVA:

H_0: Each ranking within measurements is equally likely.

H_a: At least one of the measurements produces different rankings than other measurements.

Select the level of significance from among .10, .05, .01, and .001.

As in the other nonparametric approaches, the statistic is calculated using ranked data. The researcher then compares the calculated p-value to the alpha and decides whether or not the null hypothesis may be rejected. Like with one-way repeated measures ANOVA, the significant results in Friedman's ANOVA only tell you that the measurements differ. Further investigation should be completed using the Wilcoxon signed-rank test.

To conduct Friedman's ANOVA in SPSS, you will go to Analyze > Nonparametric tests > Legacy dialogs > K related samples, as shown in **Figure 13-12**. In the Tests for Several Related Samples dialogue box, you will move variables to be paired into "Test Variables" in order by clicking the corresponding arrow buttons in the middle (see **Figure 13-13**). You will notice that "Friedman" is checked by default under "Test Type," and this option will produce statistics of Friedman's ANOVA. Notice that you can request descriptive statistics by clicking on the "Statistics" button and checking "Descriptives" in the Several Related Samples dialogue box as shown in **Figure 13-14**. Clicking "Continue" and then "OK" will then produce the output. Example output is shown in **Table 13-8**.

Figure 13-12

Selecting Friedman's ANOVA in SPSS.

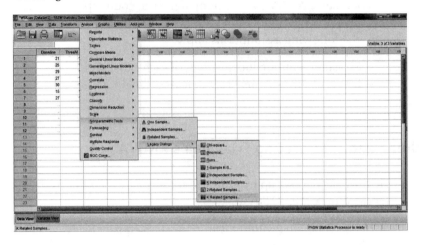

Figure 13-13

Defining variables in Friedman's ANOVA in SPSS.

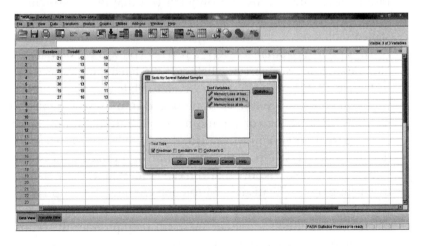

Figure 13-14

Requesting descriptives for Friedman's ANOVA in SPSS.

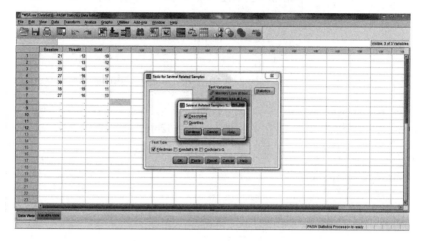

Reporting Friedman's ANOVA

When reporting Friedman's ANOVA results, you should report the size of corresponding statistics and associated *p*-value. You should also report medians of repeated measurements so that the readers will know how the sample statistic is different.

The following is a sample report from our example:

- Memory loss of participants did not significantly differ among the three different time periods, χ^2 (2) = 12.29, p = .002. Wilcoxon signed-rank tests with Bonferroni correction were used to follow up the significant findings and all effects are determined to be significant at .0167. The results indicated that memory loss at baseline was not significantly different from that at 3 months after music therapy, z = −1.61, p = .107, and at 6 months after music therapy, z = −2.37, p = .018. However, memory loss at 3 months after music therapy also did not differ from that at 6 months after music therapy, z = −2.41, p = .016.

Table	
13-8	**Example Output of Friedman's ANOVA in SPSS**

Descriptive Statistics

	N	Mean	Std. Deviation	Minimum	Maximum
Memory loss at baseline	7	26.00	5.132	15	30
Memory loss at 3 months after music therapy	7	22.71	2.928	19	26
Memory loss at 6 months after music therapy	7	10.00	2.582	7	14

Ranks

	Mean Rank
Memory loss at baseline	2.86
Memory loss at 3 months after music therapy	2.14
Memory loss at 6 months after music therapy	1.00

Test Statistics[a]

N	7
Chi-square	12.286
df	2
Asymp. sig.	.002

[a] Friedman's test

SUMMARY

Nonparametric tests are counterparts of parametric tests and can be used in situations where the assumptions of parametric tests are violated or the sample sizes are small. Most nonparametric tests analyze the rank of the data, not the actual raw data.

When there are two independent groups to be compared and the assumptions are violated, either Mann–Whitney tests or Wilcoxon rank-sum tests can be used. If the assumptions are violated when there are two related measurements to be compared, Wilcoxon signed-rank tests can be used.

With three independent groups in comparison when the assumptions are violated, Kruskal–Wallis tests can be used instead of one-way ANOVA. Friedman's ANOVA is applicable instead of one-way repeated measures ANOVA when there are three or more related measurements in comparison.

Critical Thinking Questions

1. List and explain some situations in which nonparametric tests can be used.
2. Suppose that a friend of yours is pleased that the results of a Kruskal–Wallis test he ran as part of his dissertation turned out to be statistically significant at alpha = .05. He followed up this significant result with 15 Mann–Whitney tests and found out the results were also statistically significant at alpha = .05.
   a. Briefly explain to your friend why he needs to exercise caution in interpreting his one significant finding.
   b. If the one test your friend found to be significant had a p-value of .009, would this test have been statistically significant if he had used a Bonferroni-adjusted alpha? Why or why not?

Self-Quiz www

1. True or false: Nonparametric tests are preferred over parametric tests when the assumption(s) of parametric tests is violated.
2. What is the nonparametric counterpart of one-way ANOVA?
   a. Mann–Whitney test
   b. Kruskal–Wallis test
   c. Wilcoxon signed-rank test
   d. None of the above

3. True or false: Nonparametric tests can be used even when the data are not continuously measured.

4. True or false: When two independent groups are compared with normality assumption being violated, we can use Wilcoxon signed-rank test.

REFERENCE

Kneipp, S. M., Kairalla, J. A., Lutz, B. L., Pereira, D., Hall, A. G., Flocks, J., . . . Schwartz, T. (2011). Public health nursing case management for women receiving Temporary Assistance for Needy Families: A randomized controlled trial using community-based participatory research. *American Journal of Public Health, 101*(9), 1759–1768.

14

Categorical Data Analysis

Learning Objectives

The principal goal of this chapter is to help you develop an understanding of how to conduct and interpret findings from an analysis of association between two categorical variables. This chapter will prepare you to:

- Understand and explain the concepts of the chi-square test procedure
- Evaluate the assumptions of the chi-square statistic
- Understand the results from the chi-square test, as well as power of the effect
- Report the findings in APA style correctly
- Understand how and when associations of categorical variables are used in evidence-based practice

Key Terms

Categorical data	Fisher's exact test
Chi-square test	Odds ratio
Contingency tables	Phi and Cramer's V
Crosstab analysis	Relative risk

TESTS OF ASSOCIATION USING ORDINAL AND NOMINAL DATA

We are often interested in relationships between variables. When variables are measured at the interval or ratio level (also called continuous variables), we use Pearson's r to determine significance. However, we do not always have control over the measurement of variables, and some variables that we are interested in can only be measured at the ordinal or nominal level.

For example, we might be interested in variables such as blood type (A, B, O, or AB), response level to treatment (recovery, disability, death), or ethnicity. These data are measured at the nominal or ordinal level and do not lend themselves to arithmetic analyses. These types of data are often called **categorical data**. We saw in Chapter 5 that a categorical variable may be examined through a frequency analysis (for example, counting the number of times the patient recovers), but a frequency analysis does not help us understand the relationship between two or more categorical variables. **Crosstab analysis** is a simple extension of frequency analysis and allows us to examine the association between two or more categorical variables in terms of joint frequencies. As both variables are categorical, descriptive statistics of mean and standard deviation do not make sense. Instead, we analyze the frequency and/or percentage/proportion to answer questions about associations between variables.

Researchers may examine the associations between categorical variables to understand health and disease in relation to socioeconomic factors, race and ethnicity, geographical location, etc. A researcher might ask a question such as, "Is there a relationship between where a patient resides (urban or rural) and his health status (excellent, good, fair, or poor)?" In this case, a variable, place of residence, is nominal level data and has two possible choices; the other variable is ordinal and has four possible choices. Similarly, the nurse in an advanced practice or leadership role might ask quality improvement questions such as, "What is the relationship between the presence or absence of a patient navigator (a nurse who helps patients negotiate complex health problems and treatment) and patient satisfaction (high, moderate, or low)?"

Interpretation of the results of these types of studies must be made with an understanding of the strengths and limitations of each approach and the underlying assumptions of the statistical analysis. Advanced practice nurses and nurse leaders must be able to recognize what variables are being studied, what hypotheses are proposed, and the level of measurement for each variable; they must also evaluate the appropriateness of the statistic chosen for the analysis.

Case Study

Aiken, L. H., Clarke, S. P., Cheung, R. B., Sloane, D. M., & Silver, J. H. (2003). Educational levels of hospital nurses and surgical patient mortality. *Journal of the American Medical Association, 290*(12), 1617–1623.

In 2003, Dr. Linda Aiken and colleagues published a study in the *Journal of the American Medical Association* examining the relationship between the composition of registered nurses (diploma, associate degree, and baccalaureate) and mortality in surgical patients. Aiken et al. hypothesized that a higher proportion of baccalaureate degree nurses in any given staffing mix in any given hospital would be associated with a reduction in the mortality rates of patients undergoing surgery. The research team conducted a cross-sectional descriptive study with a nonrandom sample of hospitals and volunteer sample of nurses in Pennsylvania. Because under these circumstances the independent and dependent variables could not be assumed to be distributed normally, the researchers used adjusted mortality rates and odds ratios in a predictive model to test the hypothesis.

The researchers reported the results in terms of an adjusted risk ratio for mortality and an odds ratio to estimate the magnitude of effect of the proportion of baccalaureate-prepared nurses on failure to rescue (when serious complications of surgery occur). The results suggest that as the proportion of baccalaureate nurses increases, the risk of mortality falls, and that with each 10% increase in baccalaureate nurses there is a 5% reduction in mortality and failure to rescue.

Aiken's study is a good example of when to use analyses of the association between frequencies of categorical variables measured at the nominal or ordinal level. The study results are important in this case as a strong rationale for increasing the proportion of baccalaureate-prepared nurses in hospitals. However, if Aiken and her colleagues had not chosen the correct statistical analyses, the findings would have been subject to serious criticism and taken less seriously.

CHI-SQUARE (χ^2) TEST

Chi-square test is the simplest method to analyze both variables that are measured on the categorical level. Note that the chi-square test is a type of nonparametric test, since the data are measured at the nominal or ordinal level, and therefore the distributional assumption will not be met. In the analysis, SPSS first creates a crosstab between the two variables and then analyzes the frequencies for a possible association. The following are example questions that can be addressed with a chi-square test:

- Is there an association between disease and a factor?
- Is there a difference on preference between two hospitals according to gender?
- Is whether or not a person smokes related to whether a person drinks coffee?
- Is satisfaction level related to types of health insurance coverage?

A **contingency table** shows the frequency distribution of the two categorical variables, and the chi-square test can be used to test the relationship between variables for any contingency table that is 2 × 2 (i.e., both variables are dichotomous at either the nominal or ordinal level of measurement) or larger in size. An example of a 2 × 2 table may be found in **Table 14-1**. Note that in this example there are two variables, age and antihistamine use, and each has two choices: for age, over or less than 30 years, and for antihistamine use, use or do not use. The 2 × 2 refers to the number of variables being analyzed simultaneously. As long as there is an adequate sample size, the number of variables is unlimited. A 3 × 3 table might be an analysis of health status (poor, good, excellent) by income (low, middle, and high).

Table			
14-1	**Example Data for Chi-Square Test**		
	Do Not Use Antihistamines	**Use Antihistamines**	**Total**
Younger than 30	105	32	137
Older than 30	72	9	81
Total	177	41	218

Assumptions

As the chi-square test is a type of nonparametric test, it does not make distributional assumptions. However, the following assumptions apply:

- All observations are independent.
- Expected count or cases in each cell should be greater than 1, and no more than 20% of cells should be less than 5.

Doing and Interpreting Chi-Square Tests

First, we need to set up hypotheses to test association between two categorical variables. They can be written as follows:

H_0: There is no association between the two categorical variables.

H_a: There is an association between the two categorical variables.

We must select the level of significance from among .10, .05, .01, and .001.

The test statistic is calculated by the following formula:

$$\chi^2 = \sum \frac{(Observed\ frequency\ -\ Expected\ frequency)^2}{Expected\ frequency}$$

where the expected frequency is found by dividing the product of the raw total frequency and column total frequency with the grand

Table			
14-2	**Example Data for Chi-Square Test with Expected Frequency**		
	Do Not Use Antihistamines	**Use Antihistamines**	**Total**
Younger than 30	105(111.23)	32(25.77)	137
Older than 30	72(65.77)	9(15.23)	81
Total	177	41	218

total frequency. The statistic can be conceptualized as the difference between the observed frequencies and expected frequencies in each cell of the contingency table. Let us consider an example where a researcher is interested in examining whether one age group is more prone to use antihistamines than another. Refer to **Table 14-2** for an example data set.

The numbers inside the contingency table represent the observed frequency. For example, there are 105 people who are younger than 30 years and do not use antihistamines, 32 who are younger than 30 years and use antihistamines, 72 who are older than 30 years and do not use antihistamines, and 9 who are older than 30 years and use antihistamines. We need to calculate the expected frequency to be able to compute the chi-square statistic as shown in the previous equation, and it is the ratio of the raw total frequency multiplied by the column total frequency over the grand total frequency. For example, the expected frequency of all four cells will be the following:

$$Expected\ frequency_{younger\ than\ 30\ who\ do\ not\ use\ antihistamine} = \frac{137 \times 177}{218} = 111.23$$

$$Expected\ frequency_{younger\ than\ 30\ who\ use\ antihistamine} = \frac{137 \times 41}{218} = 25.77$$

$$Expected\ frequency_{older\ than\ 30\ who\ do\ not\ use\ antihistamine} = \frac{81 \times 177}{218} = 65.77$$

$$Expected\ frequency_{older\ than\ 30\ who\ use\ antihistamine} = \frac{81 \times 41}{218} = 15.23$$

Then, the chi-square statistic is

$$\chi^2 = \frac{(105 - 111.23)^2}{111.23} + \frac{(32 - 25.77)^2}{25.77} + \frac{(72 - 65.77)^2}{65.77} + \frac{(9 - 15.23)^2}{15.23} = 4.99$$

Once the statistic is computed, it is compared with the critical value and we make a decision to reject or not reject the null hypothesis. We reject when the statistic is larger than the critical value, similar to comparing the associated *p*-value with the statistic with alpha.

For our example, the critical value with alpha of .05 is equal to 3.841 as shown in Appendix C. Therefore, our decision is to reject the null hypothesis and to conclude that age (being older or younger than 30 years) is associated with antihistamine use.

To conduct a chi-square test in SPSS, you will go to Analyze > Descriptive Statistics > Crosstabs as shown in **Figure 14-1**. In the Crosstabs dialogue box, insert one of the variables into the "Row(s)" box and the other into the "Column(s)" box (**Figure 14-2**). Click on the "Statistics" button, which allows you to conduct various statistical tests, but notice that none are checked by default in the Crosstab Statistics dialogue box. Click on "Chi-square," as shown in **Figure 14-3**. This will perform the actual test and produce the results of significance testing. Clicking "Continue" and then "OK" will then produce the output. The example output is shown in **Table 14-3**.

Figure 14-1

Selecting a chi-square test in SPSS.

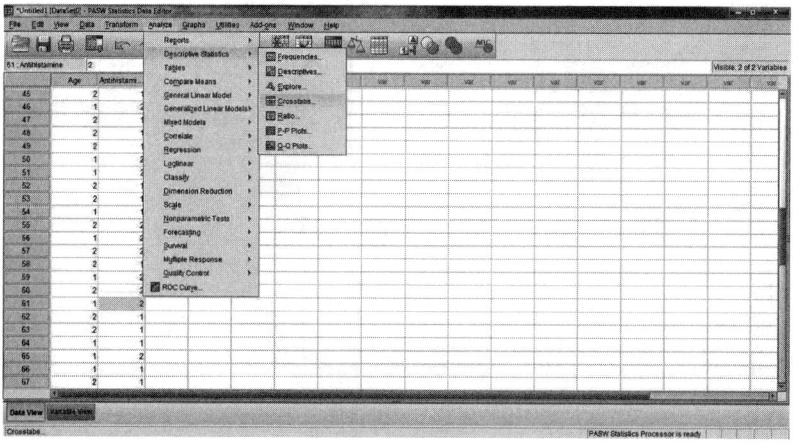

Figure 14-2

Defining variables in chi-square tests in SPSS.

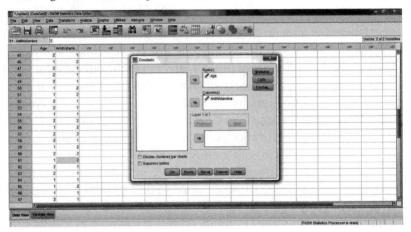

Reporting Chi-Square Tests

When reporting chi-square tests results, you should report the size of corresponding chi-square statistics with its associated degrees of freedom and the p-value. The following is a sample report from our example:

- There was a significant association between the age group and whether or not they use antihistamines, $\chi^2 (1) = 23.73, p = .000$.

Figure 14-3

Checking options in chi-square tests in SPSS.

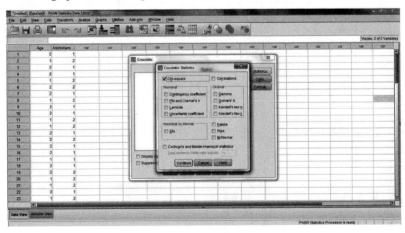

Table	
14-3	**Example Output of Chi-Square Tests in SPSS**

Case Processing Summary

	Cases					
	Valid		Missing		Total	
	N	Percent	N	Percent	N	Percent
Age * antihistamine	74	100.0%	0	.0%	74	100.0%

Age * Antihistamine Crosstabulation
Count

		Antihistamine		
		Do Not Use Antihistamine	Use Antihistamine	Total
Age	Younger than 30	8	27	35
	Older than 30	31	8	39
Total		39	35	74

Chi-Square Tests

	Value	df	Asymp. Sig. (2-Sided)	Exact Sig. (2-Sided)	Exact Sig. (1-Sided)
Pearson chi-square	23.732[a]	1	.000		
Continuity correction[b]	21.514	1	.000		
Likelihood ratio	25.162	1	.000		
Fisher's exact test				.000	.000
Linear-by-linear association	23.411	1	.000		
N of valid cases	74				

[a] 0 cells (.0%) have expected count less than 5. The minimum expected count is 16.55.
[b] Computed only for a 2 × 2 table

(continued)

Table			
14-3	**Continued**		
	Symmetric Measures		
		Value	**Approx. Sig.**
Nominal by nominal	Phi	−.566	.000
	Cramer's V	.566	.000
N of valid cases		74	

In this case, the degrees of freedom are equal to $(r - 1) \times (c - 1)$, where r is the number of rows and c is the number of columns in the contingency table. Therefore, we get $(2 - 1) \times (2 - 1) = 1$.

FISHER'S EXACT TEST

One of the assumptions of chi-square test was that the expected count in all cells should be greater than 1 and no more than 20% of cells should have a count of less than 5. The chi-square test becomes unstable (a less reliable and less valid analytic tool) when this assumption is violated (i.e., expected count in any cell is small). Fisher (1922), the famous statistician, developed **Fisher's exact test** in order to resolve this problem. Note that Fisher's exact test should only be used with 2×2 contingency tables when the sample size is small enough that the assumption can be violated. As we have seen in Table 14-3, the output of the chi-square test reports additional statistics, including Fisher's exact test. Let us consider the following output where we slightly modify the data so that some cells have an expected frequency of less than 5. That output is shown in **Table 14-4**. Notice that the cells for people who are younger than 30 and do not use antihistamines, and for people who are older than 30 and use antihistamines, have expected frequencies of less than 5, which violates the assumption. Therefore, the result of Fisher's exact test should be reported instead of that of chi-square test. In our example, both p-values are less than the alpha of .05, so the results are significant anyway.

Table	
14-4	**Example Output When Some Cells Have an Expected Frequency of Less Than 5**

Age * Antihistamine Crosstabulation
Count

		Antihistamine		
		Do Not Use Antihistamine	**Use Antihistamine**	**Total**
Age	Younger than 30	1	7	8
	Older than 30	9	4	13
Total		10	11	21

Chi-Square Tests

	Value	**df**	**Asymp. Sig. (2-Sided)**	**Exact Sig. (2-Sided)**	**Exact Sig. (1-Sided)**
Pearson chi-square	6.390[a]	1	.011		
Continuity correction[b]	4.318	1	.038		
Likelihood ratio	6.988	1	.008		
Fisher's exact test				.024	.017
Linear-by-linear association	6.086	1	.014		
N of valid cases	21				

[a] 2 cells (50.0%) have expected count less than 5. The minimum expected count is 3.81.
[b] Computed only for a 2 × 2 table

PHI AND CRAMER'S V

When "Chi-square" is checked in the Crosstabs Statistics dialogue box, it calculates the statistic with its associated *p*-value and tells us whether the two categorical variables are related. However, the significant results of chi-square only indicate that the variables are related and do not tell anything about the strength of relationship. In the

Figure 14-4

Choosing Phi and Cramer's V in chi-square test in SPSS.

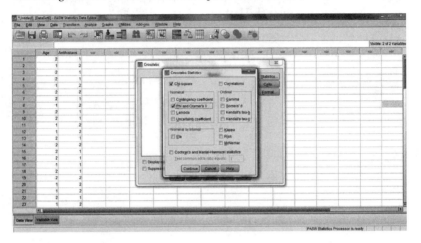

Crosstab Statistics box, there are two statistics we can calculate and report when the strength of association is of interest; they are **Phi and Cramer's V**. Let us click on the "Statistics" button and check "Phi and Cramer's V," as shown in **Figure 14-4**, to calculate measures for the strength of association between the two variables.

Phi is used when both variables are dichotomous, but Cramer's V should be used when one of the two categorical variables is measured on more than two categories. Phi (ϕ) ranges between -1 and 1, while Cramer's V ranges between 0 and 1; the general rule for correlation coefficients can be used to interpret them (as discussed in Chapter 9). As the coefficient approaches 0, the association between the two categorical variables is weak, while it is stronger as it approaches 1. Negative and positive signs will indicate whether the association is a positive or negative relationship. Note that these statistical tests can also be used as a measure of effect size. Reporting of these statistics can be added after the associated p-value with chi-square tests statistics. Here is a sample report:

- There was a significant association between the age group and antihistamine use, χ^2 (1) = 8.24, $p < .01$, $\phi = -.63$.

Table			
14-5	**The Data for Smoking and Lung Cancer**		
	Lung Cancer	**No Lung Cancer**	**Total**
Smokers	86	48	134
Nonsmokers	23	71	94
Total	109	119	228

Relative Risk and Odds Ratio

When categorical data are collected in 2 × 2 contingency tables, there are other measures of effect size than Phi and Cramer's V. Two common ones are **relative risk** (RR) and **odds ratio** (OR). The RR is defined as the measure of the *risk of an outcome* (e.g., disease or death) occurring when exposed to a risk factor, while the OR is defined as the *ratio of an outcome* (e.g., disease or death) occurring when exposed to a risk factor. For example, the RR is the probability a patient who smokes will develop lung cancer relative to that of a nonsmoking patient, and the OR is the odds of a patient who smokes developing lung cancer divided by the odds of a nonsmoking patient developing lung cancer. Note that both measures can be calculated and interpreted only for 2 × 2 contingency tables.

Let us take the following example where an association between smoking and lung cancer is examined; the data are shown in **Table 14-5**. Then, the RR is calculated as follows:

$$RR = \frac{P(an\ outcome\ occuring\ when\ exposed\ to\ a\ risk\ factor)}{P(an\ outcome\ occurring\ when\ not\ exposed\ to\ a\ risk\ factor)}$$

$$= \frac{\frac{86}{134}}{\frac{23}{94}}$$

$$= 2.62$$

and the OR is calculated as follows:

$$OR = \frac{\textit{Odds of an outcome occuring when exposed to a risk factor}}{\textit{Odds of an outcome occurring when not exposed to a risk factor}}$$

$$= \frac{\dfrac{86}{48}}{\dfrac{23}{71}}$$

$$= 5.53$$

Interpreting both the RR and the OR can be done in the same manner. If either the RR or OR is equal to 1, it implies that the risk or odds of the two groups are the same in terms of an outcome occurring. If that was the case in our example, it would mean that it does not matter whether or not you smoke in getting lung cancer. If either the RR or OR is greater than 1, it implies that there is a positive association between the outcome occurring and an exposure to a risk factor; therefore, an exposure to a risk factor will increase the occurrence of an outcome. For our example, you will be 2.63 (or 5.53 for odds ratio) times more likely to get lung cancer if you smoke. If either the RR or OR is less than 1, it implies that there is a negative association between the outcome occurring and an exposure to a risk factor. Note that a corresponding confidence interval should also be reported when both the RR and the OR are reported. An example report for the data in Table 14-5 is shown below:

- There was a significant association between smoking and getting lung cancer, $\chi^2 (1) = 34.92$, $p = .000$. Odds ratio was also computed for this data and indicates that the odds of getting lung cancer were 5.53 times (95% CI: 3.07, 9.96) higher for a smoking person than a nonsmoking person.

From the previous example, we saw the RR and the OR could produce different results. So, which one should we use? Both measures examine an association between exposure to a risk factor and the occurrence of an outcome, but they are not the same measures. The RR measures whether an exposure to a risk factor makes a difference in the occurrence of the outcome, whereas the OR measures whether there is a difference in an exposure to a risk factor in those with and without the occurrence of an outcome.

Often times, the RR is an easier and more interpretable measure of an association, but the OR has been more widely used in statistics, particularly with logistic regression in clinical studies. The OR is commonly used for case-control studies, in which noncondition and condition groups are compared in an attempt to identify factors that may contribute to an outcome, whereas the RR is commonly used in cohort studies (i.e., longitudinal analysis of risk factors) or randomized controlled trials.

SUMMARY

The chi-square test is the preferred method to investigate an association between two categorical variables. Assumptions include independence of observations and adequate sample size for each cell; therefore, it is a nonparametric test.

In cases where any cell contains a frequency of less than 5 in 2×2 contingency tables, Fisher's exact test can be used and reported instead of chi-square test, since the chi-square becomes unstable with a small sample size.

The significant results of chi-square only indicate that the variables are related, so we may need a different measure of strength of association. Phi and Cramer's V are such measures. Phi is reported for 2×2 contingency tables, whereas Cramer's V is reported for larger contingency tables.

Relative risk (RR) and odds ratios (ORs) can also be computed and reported as effect sizes. The RR is defined as the measure of the risk of an outcome (e.g., disease or death) occurring when exposed to a risk factor, and the OR is defined as the ratio of an outcome (e.g., disease or death) occurring when exposed to a risk factor. Both should be reported with their associated confidence interval.

Critical Thinking Questions www

1. Explain why the chi-square test is part of the family of nonparametric tests.
2. A researcher found that there is a significant association between gender and pain level (low vs. high), and the associated Phi measure was .30. How would the researcher interpret this measure? Explain.

3. Briefly describe a potential study in your field where you might use a chi-square test.
   a. Provide a one- or two-sentence description of the study, e.g., nature of the subjects/participants, purpose, etc.
   b. State the research question that would be answered by a chi-square test.
   c. Describe the variables to be used for the chi-square test.
   d. Indicate what a statistically significant chi-square test in this particular study would tell you.

Self-Quiz www

1. True or false: A significant chi-square test result will tell us that the two variables are associated and how strong a relationship is.
2. Which of the following statistics should be reported when any cell has expected frequency of less than 5 in a 2×2 contingency table?
   a. Chi-square
   b. Likelihood ratio
   c. Fisher's exact test
   d. Linear-by-linear association
3. True or false: Cramer's V is more appropriate measure for the strength of association than Phi when the size of contingency table is 2×2.
4. True or false: The relative risk is used with a cohort study, whereas the odds ratio is used for a case-control study.

REFERENCES

Aiken, L. H., Clarke, S. P., Cheung, R. B., Sloane, D. M., & Silver, J. H. (2003). Educational levels of hospital nurses and surgical patient mortality. *Journal of the American Medical Association, 290*(12), 1617–1623.

Fisher, R. A. (1922). On the interpretation of χ^2 from contingency tables, and the calculation of P. *Journal of the Royal Statistical Society, 85*(1), 87–94. doi: 10.2307/2340521

15 Common Statistical Mistakes

Learning Objectives

The principal goal of this chapter is to discuss commonly made statistical mistakes and how these can be avoided. This chapter will prepare you to:

- Understand the common types of statistical mistakes
- Recognize the consequences of making statistical mistakes and avoid the statistical mistakes outlined here

INTRODUCTION

In this text we have discussed why nurses in advanced practice or leadership and management positions need to have a working understanding of basic statistical tools and how these help to apply research to practice and conduct quality improvement projects, program evaluation, and other projects that generate numerical data. All projects are designed and carried out by fallible human beings, and mistakes are sometimes made. More often, project findings are limited by the decisions that designers have made in the face of complex systems. For example, we have seen that the most robust statistical tests assume random sampling to ensure a normal distribution of the variable in the sample. However, many researchers and project leaders find that random sampling is not feasible in the environment in which the project is being carried out. All studies and projects have flaws and limitations. In a good report, the author has assessed these limitations and explicitly states them in the discussion of the findings. As a consumer of such reports, you must decide if the study findings are still useful on balance with the flaws. As a study or project leader, you want to develop a design that is as strong as possible given the known limitations in carrying out the work.

Statistical mistakes can occur at various stages of a study or project. Such errors include poor sampling strategy, inaccurate data entry, mispresenting a graph, or choosing the wrong statistical test for the proposed research questions. The goal of this chapter is to discuss the most commonly made statistical mistakes in order to acknowledge and avoid them.

MISTAKE #1: OVERLOOKING THE IMPORTANCE OF CHECKING ASSUMPTIONS

Each statistical test has its own assumptions. For example, let us consider a researcher who is interested in examining the differences among four cultural groups on patient satisfaction . The researcher will choose a one-way analysis of variance (ANOVA), and ANOVA requires the following three assumptions to be met:

- The sample data follows a normal distribution.
- Observations are independent.
- The variances across different groups are homogeneous.

However, these assumptions may be ignored or the researcher may deliberately choose to violate the assumptions and carry out the statistical test. Keselman et al. (1998) reviewed articles in 17 journals and found that researchers rarely verify that the required assumptions are met in the data, and this criticism unfortunately still continues. ANOVA compares the means of each group, but the means of groups will be biased when the distribution of the variable is not normal. Therefore, such results may not be trustworthy or may be limited.

In the case of a violation of these assumptions, a researcher should try a remedy such as a transformation to see if it helps to correct a violation. If not, he or she should try nonparametric tests. Nonparametric tests are generally lower in power and precision than that of their parametric counterparts, but they do not have any of the parametric assumptions. The lower power results from calculating statistics with rank-ordered data instead of the raw data; thus, there are not distributional assumptions. As such, they should be used over parametric tests in cases of assumption violation. Remember that the violation of assumptions will lead to biased results.

MISTAKE #2: ARBITRARILY SELECTING THE SAMPLE SIZE

As we have discussed in Chapter 7, there is a close relationship among type I error, type II error, sample size, and the power of the hypotheses testing. When sample size is small, there is a higher chance of committing a type II error, which results in decreased power; in other words, you will not be able to reject the null hypothesis when you should. Therefore, it makes sense to perform an a priori power analysis to make sure that the test has enough power to detect a significant effect with an adequate sample size. Remember that a small sample size will decrease statistical power in detecting a significant effect.

MISTAKE #3: DELETING MISSING DATA WITHOUT JUSTIFICATION

In any survey design, there are many reasons for data to be missing. For example, a patient may have simply decided not to participate or may have been lost to follow-up during the longitudinal study period. As missing data can introduce bias into the analyses, the researcher must make decisions on what to do with missing data.

It is not uncommon to see that the researcher has deleted cases that include these missing data, but this also introduces bias into the analyses. An important question to ask before deleting missing data is, "Are patients who participated different from those who did not participate (dropped out)?" If they are not different, the deletion may not cause a serious distortion in the results. However, this distortion may become serious when those cases deleted from the analysis are different from those remaining; we lose information from those who did not participate or died, and the loss of information introduces a bias into the results.

Another important question is whether the amount of missing data is small or large, as compared to the total sample size. If it is only a small fraction of the sample size, then the deletion of missing data may not be a big concern. However, it will be an inappropriate action to take if the amount of missing data is large. Again, there is an issue of losing information, so you should not delete the missing data only because they are missing. Rather, you should make sure they are not different than the rest in the data.

MISTAKE #4: MISPRESENTATION OF THE DATA

One common mistake is the failure to present the data in the most accurate format. Accurate display and reporting of data and statistical analyses is an important part of the statistical results to be reported. Consider **Figure 15-1** as an example of how the data could be mispresented and possibly cause distortion of readers' understanding. The data represent the average number of admissions to an emergency room per month, and the two graphs seem to present different data. However, you will notice that the data are the same (the raw data are within a 24–26 range), but the vertical scales of the two graphs are different. Figure 15-1a shows the data with full bars showing not much of a difference across months. On the other hand, Figure 15-1b only shows the top of the bars, which seem to be in a much larger range. Is it correct to conclude that there was a large difference over the months in terms of the number of admissions to an emergency room? How the data are presented can lead to distortions.

Figure 15-1

Example of data mispresentation using a graph.

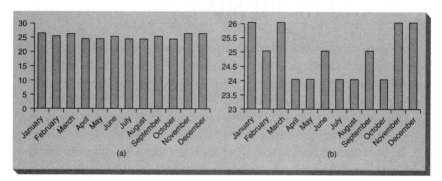

Also consider the following statement: *The number of residents in our nursing home has dropped by 25%, but the average number of falls this month is 33, up from 26 in the last month. We had about a 50% jump in the average number of falls this month, so we need to investigate the cause of it.* Is this an accurate conclusion to make? If the nursing home has not experienced a change in the number of residents, then, yes, it may be a correct statement. However, the number of residents has actually dropped over the year, making a conclusion about the average number of falls without considering the number of residents misleading. Remember that you have to be careful with the way data are presented!

MISTAKE #5: CORRELATION IMPLIES CAUSATION

A correlation coefficient is a measure of the relationship between the variables and tells us whether two or more variables of interest are related with each other. For example, a correlation coefficient of +.59 between age and systolic blood pressure (SBP) means that age and SBP are positively related (i.e., as the age of a person goes up or down, his/her SBP increases or decreases, respectively). However, this does not necessarily imply that one of the two variables causes the change in the other variable, since a correlation coefficient *only* indicates a relationship or association between the variables. Remember that correlation does not imply causation!

MISTAKE #6: CONFUSING STATISTICAL SIGNIFICANCE WITH PRACTICAL OR CLINICAL IMPORTANCE

We are familiar with this point after discussing effect sizes in Chapter 7. Statistical significance alone does not tell us about how much of an effect was present and how important the size of the effect is in clinical practice. Statistical nonsignificance can still have practical importance. For instance, a researcher may find that a new treatment produces a clinically significant improvement, but does not produce statistically significant results. On the other hand, statistical significance may not have practical importance. Remember that statistical significance and practical importance are not related!

MISTAKE #7: EXTRAPOLATING A REGRESSION PREDICTION LINE

In a regression analysis, we find a line of the best fit for the data and try to predict an outcome variable using information from an independent variable. However, this prediction should remain only within the measurement range of the independent variable used in fitting the line of the best fit. If we use this prediction line outside of this initial range, we do not know how good a prediction it will be, as those values outside of the initial range were not used in the process of finding the line of the best fit. Remember: Extrapolation is dangerous!

MISTAKE #8: RUNNING MULTIPLE TESTS SIMULTANEOUSLY

It is common that a researcher wants to compare two or more groups on multiple dependent variables to see if there exist any group differences on dependent variables. However, running multiple tests simultaneously raises a problem. As discussed in Chapter 7, a researcher should predetermine the level of significance, indicating how much type I error he or she is comfortable in making. Let us assume that the researcher decided to use .05 on the tests. If a single test is conducted, the level of significance stays at .05, and this is compared to the p-value in making a statistical decision. However, the level of significance is not equal to .05 when the multiple tests are performed; instead, it gets inflated with the increased numbers of tests.

For any given set of statistical tests, the inflated type I error will be:

$$\alpha_{\text{Inflated}} = 1 - (1 - \alpha_{\text{prespecified}})^n$$

where α_{Inflated} is the type I error inflated after conducting multiple tests, $\alpha_{\text{prespecified}}$ is the prespecified/desired type I error, and n is the number of tests. As you can see, the type I error will be inflated more as more tests are being conducted. For example, say you want to run three tests, each at a type I error of .05. Then, the type I error is inflated to

$$\alpha_{\text{Inflated}} = 1 - (1 - .05)^3 = .1426$$

Therefore, you should either correct this inflation using Bonferroni adjustment or use a better design that controls for the inflated type I error problem—for example, you can do one-way ANOVA instead of a series of independent t-tests. Note that you may follow the suggestion of the APA *Publication Manual* (2010) for the reporting of exact p-values in reported results and allow the readers to interpret the reported results. Remember that there is an increased risk of committing higher type I error with running multiple tests simultaneously.

MISTAKE #9: CONFUSING PAIRED DATA AND NONPAIRED DATA

Nonpaired data are those that have unique subjects in each of the groups (i.e., there are no overlapping subjects across the groups), whereas paired data are nested within the same group of subjects. When a group of subjects gets different treatments and are to give ratings on each of them, for example, the data are paired or nested within the same group of people. Sometimes, the term "different treatments" confuses students' thinking and this leads them to perform a nonpaired data analysis. However, this would be incorrect since the data are still nested within the same group of people, and thus are paired. Gender differences on the attitudes toward healthcare reform and the attitudes towards lesbian and gay population by staff and administrative nurses are some clear examples of nonpaired data. Remember that there is a clear distinction between nonpaired data and paired data!

MISTAKE #10: SELECTING INAPPROPRIATE STATISTICAL TESTS

We have emphasized the importance of correctly identifying the level of measurements of a variable because it directs us to the appropriate statistical test to answer the proposed research questions. If you are interested in examining a relationship between two categorical variables, like gender and opinion (i.e., against and in favor), you would run a chi-square test of independence. However, you would run a one-way ANOVA if opinion is measured on a continuous level of measurement using a Likert scale instrument. Therefore, you should pay close attention to the level of measurement and determine which test will be the most appropriate.

Another common mistake is to perform parametric statistical tests even when the data violate the test's assumptions, such as the normality of a variable. All parametric tests assume that the variable is normally distributed, and the results from these tests cannot be trustworthy if this assumption is violated. For example, the use of parametric tests for non-normally distributed data may provide a significant effect. However, this is more likely a result of type I error. As nonparametric tests are more powerful when the assumption is violated than parametric tests, it is right to use nonparametric tests in this situation. Remember that the results using an incorrect statistical test are nothing more than garbage.

SUMMARY

Statistics is an important tool for researchers to answer their research questions. However, they may not produce reliable results when possible sources of mistakes are not carefully considered and addressed beforehand.

Some of the most commonly made mistakes include, but are not limited to, overlooking the importance of checking assumptions, arbitrarily selecting the sample size, deleting missing data without justification, mispresenting the data, implying causation from correlation, confusing statistical significance with practical importance, extrapolating a regression prediction line, running multiple tests simultaneously, confusing paired data and nonpaired data, and performing inappropriate statistical tests.

These are examples of mistakes that can be avoided with care in designing the study. Remember that these errors will introduce bias and produce unreliable results.

Critical Thinking Questions

1. Think of an example that you may want to study using an independent samples *t*-test. Explain why the violation of normality assumption will bias the results.
2. Explain why the violation of assumptions can lead to a false result.
3. Selection of sample size is important in the design stage of any study. Explain why.

Self-Quiz

1. True or false: When parametric tests are used, one should check the normality of the variable of interest before conducting the proposed test.
2. What is the consequence of running multiple tests without any adjustment?
   a. Inflating type II error
   b. Inflating type I error
   c. Increasing the power of the test
   d. All of the above

REFERENCES

American Psychological Association (APA). (2010). *Publication manual of the American Psychological Association* (6th ed.). Washington, DC: Author.

Keselman, H. J., Huberty, C. J., Lix, L. M., Olejnik, S., Cribbie, R. A., Donahue, B., . . . Levin, J. R. (1998). Statistical practices of educational researchers: An analysis of their ANOVA, MANOVA and ANCOVA analyses. *Review of Educational Research, 68*(3), 350–386.

Appendix

Random Number Table

76009	57168	74931	96606	88035	76252	79871	89652	67307	79856
26196	46586	58991	46728	85684	20316	47616	39721	79743	79485
S92S2	94064	83711	50447	92640	96251	21056	92617	88231	36646
30028	31847	43969	53956	90732	54110	47468	14742	81987	93510
19371	97913	39628	79893	19300	92429	13070	34914	42268	61808
74900	53606	92806	36617	43667	97911	38719	58578	54005	21460
18579	78496	34453	92126	14126	25984	85145	75320	70084	43530
36459	36092	11685	52881	71845	85373	27316	71660	34604	97339
70598	58402	11142	72876	56030	98083	18147	47336	43413	33605
78148	44575	43186	41280	98869	97489	78276	47930	39783	81567
26023	38684	82164	94437	60156	36045	91839	93451	45574	53148
55134	49766	59890	74924	63575	77021	57934	43632	76988	36004
19106	28428	89571	78819	25600	76469	80373	87786	38186	34693
90066	35756	41368	14695	96632	62338	18160	69498	65060	81919
65617	81584	55932	39632	44126	70882	78861	81448	48806	43863
10988	62003	36376	64177	39016	52911	62190	58257	30091	17353
88063	35508	35233	89686	24129	56640	21337	29446	72289	24367
68637	40608	51395	23205	79440	97135	85570	44210	60237	15895
90778	38815	54550	40731	91659	39548	58912	49362	83173	95825
78592	11123	68508	36810	65063	57392	77253	38070	72466	96400
99922	25624	82404	31031	42521	21016	77157	36176	99162	48795
69218	83808	51580	40851	81161	78460	48920	19209	77561	27902
75956	86582	61693	93234	73403	28231	24656	94239	56485	93223
85868	93287	66407	42459	90968	11282	47238	52210	77507	63355
12337	25359	84939	49801	43486	26679	81027	56685	57427	90176
20371	62131	66138	64317	91468	57051	90662	12113	22303	47317
27738	25562	24061	57551	77807	94778	96463	26899	34947	85231
56111	33666	46012	24108	54164	45900	42391	59479	89026	41704
74507	88419	59713	27194	65096	58897	94931	44830	74676	32929
70850	56369	45292	36643	40284	32356	28244	15343	72551	72950
17360	33207	56447	81856	20240	31187	27922	56227	29793	78710
23870	10779	24046	66581	33298	16256	94458	96052	42207	93511
89744	27784	30769	93385	95432	15735	40267	48189	49353	60877
25899	12480	22089	98743	19420	81709	92885	11148	68541	86675
77693	94203	53487	97764	88670	84039	51992	70381	50293	74420
58260	63879	92028	96336	10547	50014	24554	58282	94420	21170
30625	30502	14871	44372	40590	16567	99134	46069	56147	89484
94672	65076	26146	89186	83948	94726	29571	63988	46450	36627
58097	56398	62824	56267	45593	22354	16419	48976	80420	47832
96097	44097	74065	57157	88156	29319	29809	12513	25289	74520
83661	21726	35988	24501	79316	40332	20113	52232	75386	49133
36419	16341	27562	96738	70360	35745	98043	23063	90671	90328
86208	85696	98388	50545	89204	15317	86756	65420	47321	87384
53306	79845	85217	79656	24656	48001	18644	31998	46963	35554
20955	97793	29609	53295	97993	59529	13756	95516	75988	19700
97467	32999	87897	99581	31796	65575	25925	89741	81631	31899
45541	33868	96128	30613	41180	66153	47444	54352	97051	93493
37060	67665	56556	35249	43038	38164	62423	57468	15576	63597
15131	76566	67888	21508	40056	46660	55236	39305	74347	44878
13295	53488	71906	21621	28276	99234	25352	90022	37992	74088

B How to Select the Correct Statistical Test

Variables Level of Measurements/ Distribution		Test	Example
0 IV 1 DV	Interval (ratio) and normal	One sample *t*-test	Is the average number of inpatient days different than 200,000?
	Nominal	Chi-square (goodness of fit)	Is there a **preference in the selection** of cold medicine?
1 IV (2 independent groups) 1 DV	Interval (ratio) and normal	Independent samples *t*-test	Is there a difference in the **amount of salary** nurses make by gender?
	Ordinal	Mann–Whitney *U* test	Is there a difference in **opinions on "should abortion be banned?"** (measured in 5-point Likert scale) between New Jersey and New York?
	Nominal	Chi-square (Fisher's exact)	Are the drugs (A vs. B) **effective (vs. not effective)**?
1 IV (2 dependent groups) 1 DV	Interval (ratio) and normal	Dependent samples *t*-test	Does **tumor size** decrease after the treatment?
	Ordinal	Wilcoxon signed rank test	Do epilepsy-related direct medical costs **(ERDMC)** change before and after the implantation of a vagus nerve stimulator?
	Nominal	McNemar test	Does a newly developed drug have an **effect** (effective vs. noneffective for both pre and after) on treating pneumonia?

(continued)

Variables	Level of Measurements/ Distribution	Test	Example
1 IV (more than 2 independent groups)	1 DV Interval (ratio) and normal	One-way analysis of variance (ANOVA)	Is there a difference in the **amount of salary** made by nurses with different education level (i.e., ADN, BSN, MS, and PhD)?
	Ordinal	Kruskal–Wallis *H* test	Is there a difference in **opinions on "should abortion be banned?"** (measured in 5-point Likert scale) between New York, Chicago, and Los Angeles?
1 IV (More than 2 dependent groups)	1 DV Interval (ratio) and normal	One-way repeated measures ANOVA	Is there a change/difference in systolic blood pressure (SBP) over three different time periods (e.g., now, a week later, and 2 weeks later)?
	Ordinal	Friedman test	Is there a difference in **ratings** (in 5-point Likert scale) of 10 subjects for drug A, B, and C?
1 IV (2 or more independent groups) 1 covariate	1 DV Interval (ratio) and normal Interval (ratio) and normal	Analysis of covariance (ANCOVA)	Is there a gender difference on average **sodium content level**, after adjusting for their weight?

(continued)

Variables Level of Measurements/ Distribution		Test	Example
2 or more IVs (2 or more independent groups)	1 DV Interval (ratio) and normal	Factorial ANOVA	Is there a gender difference on average **sodium content level**?
			Is there an ethnicity difference on average **sodium content level**?
			Is there an interaction effect by gender and ethnicity on average **sodium content level**?
2 or more IVs (2 or more independent groups) 1 covariate Interval (ratio) and normal	1 DV Interval (ratio) and normal	Factorial ANCOVA	Is there a gender difference on average **sodium content level**, after adjusting for their weight?
			Is there an ethnicity difference on average **sodium content level**, after adjusting for their weight?
			Is there an interaction effect by gender and ethnicity on average **sodium content level**, after adjusting for their weight?
1 or more IV(s)	2 or more DVs Interval (ratio) and normal	Multivariate analysis of variance (MANOVA)	Is there a gender difference on a combined set of DVs, **SBP and cholesterol**?

(continued)

Variables Level of Measurements/ Distribution

Variables Level of Measurements/ Distribution		Test	Example
1 or more IV(s) 1 covariate Interval (ratio) and normal	2 or more DVs Interval (ratio) and normal	Multivariate analysis of covariance (MANCOVA)	Is there a gender difference on a combined set of DVs, **SBP and cholesterol**, after adjusting for their weight?
1 IV Interval (ratio) and normal	1DV Interval (ratio) and normal	Pearson' r correlation coefficient Simple linear regression	Is age related to **SBP?** Can age predict SBP?
Ordinal	Interval (ratio) and normal	Spearman's ρ Kendall's τ	Is age (measured in 5 different age groups) related to **SBP?**
2 or more IVs Nominal and/or interval (ratio) and normal	1 DV Interval (ratio) and normal	Multiple linear regression	Can age, gender, weight, and stress predict **SBP?**
2 or more IVs Nominal and/or interval (ratio) and normal	1 DV Nominal	Logistic regression	Can age, gender, time in hospitalization, and stress predict whether a patient will **die or live?**

Note: IV = independent variable; DV= dependent variable

Appendix

C   Critical Values

Table										
C-1	The Standard Normal Distribution									

z	.00	.01	.02	.03	.04	.05	.06	.07	.08	.09
0.0	.0000	.0040	.0080	.0120	.0160	.0199	.0239	.0279	.0319	.0359
0.1	.0398	.0438	.0478	.0517	.0557	.0596	.0636	.0675	.0714	.0753
0.2	.0793	.0832	.0871	.0910	.0948	.0987	.1026	.1064	.1103	.1141
0.3	.1179	.1217	.1255	.1293	.1331	.1368	.1406	.1443	.1480	.1517
0.4	.1554	.1591	.1628	.1664	.1700	.1736	.1772	.1808	.1844	.1879
0.5	.1915	.1950	.1985	.2019	.2054	.2088	.2123	.2157	.2190	.2224
0.6	.2257	.2291	.2324	.2357	.2389	.2422	.2454	.2486	.2517	.2549
0.7	.2580	.2611	.2642	.2673	.2704	.2734	.2764	.2794	.2823	.2852
0.8	.2881	.2910	.2939	.2967	.2995	.3023	.3051	.3078	.3106	.3133
0.9	.3159	.3186	.3212	.3238	.3264	.3289	.3315	.3340	.3365	.3389
1.0	.3413	.3438	.3461	.3485	.3508	.3531	.3554	.3577	.3599	.3621
1.1	.3643	.3665	.3686	.3708	.3729	.3749	.3770	.3790	.3810	.3830
1.2	.3849	.3869	.3888	.3907	.3925	.3944	.3962	.3980	.3997	.4015
1.3	.4032	.4049	.4066	.4082	.4099	.4115	.4131	.4147	.4162	.4177
1.4	.4192	.4207	.4222	.4236	.4251	.4265	.4279	.4292	.4306	.4319
1.5	.4332	.4345	.4357	.4370	.4382	.4394	.4406	.4418	.4429	.4441
1.6	.4452	.4463	.4474	.4484	.4495	.4505	.4515	.4525	.4535	.4545
1.7	.4554	.4564	.4573	.4582	.4591	.4599	.4608	.4616	.4625	.4633
1.8	.4641	.4649	.4656	.4664	.4671	.4678	.4686	.4693	.4699	.4706
1.9	.4713	.4719	.4726	.4732	.4738	.4744	.4750	.4756	.4761	.4767
2.0	.4772	.4778	.4783	.4788	.4793	.4798	.4803	.4808	.4812	.4817
2.1	.4821	.4826	.4830	.4834	.4838	.4842	.4846	.4850	.4854	.4857
2.2	.4861	.4864	.4868	.4871	.4875	.4878	.4881	.4884	.4887	.4890
2.3	.4893	.4896	.4898	.4901	.4904	.4906	.4909	.4911	.4913	.4916
2.4	.4918	.4920	.4922	.4925	.4927	.4929	.4931	.4932	.4934	.4936
2.5	.4938	.4940	.4941	.4943	.4945	.4946	.4948	.4949	.4951	.4952
2.6	.4953	.4955	.4956	.4957	.4959	.4960	.4961	.4962	.4963	.4964
2.7	.4965	.4966	.4967	.4968	.4969	.4970	.4971	.4972	.4973	.4974
2.8	.4974	.4975	.4976	.4977	.4977	.4978	.4979	.4979	.4980	.4981
2.9	.4981	.4982	.4982	.4983	.4984	.4984	.4985	.4985	.4986	.4986
3.0	.4987	.4987	.4987	.4988	.4988	.4989	.4989	.4989	.4990	.4990

Table	The t Distribution (Values of t_α —One-Tailed Test)					
C-2						
d.f.	$t_{.100}$	$t_{.050}$	$t_{.025}$	$t_{.010}$	$t_{.005}$	**d.f.**
1	3.078	6.314	12.706	31.821	63.657	1
2	1.886	2.920	4.303	6.965	9.925	2
3	1.638	2.353	3.182	4.541	5.841	3
4	1.533	2.132	2.776	3.747	4.604	4
5	1.476	2.015	2.571	3.365	4.032	5
6	1.440	1.943	2.447	3.143	3.707	6
7	1.415	1.895	2.365	2.998	3.499	7
8	1.397	1.860	2.306	2.896	3.355	8
9	1.383	1.833	2.262	2.821	3.250	9
10	1.372	1.812	2.228	2.764	3.169	10
11	1.363	1.796	2.201	2.718	3.106	11
12	1.356	1.782	2.179	2.681	3.055	12
13	1.350	1.771	2.160	2.650	3.012	13
14	1.345	1.761	2.145	2.624	2.977	14
15	1.341	1.753	2.131	2.602	2.947	15
16	1.337	1.746	2.120	2.583	2.921	16
17	1.333	1.740	2.110	2.567	2.898	17
18	1.330	1.734	2.101	2.552	2.878	18
19	1.328	1.729	2.093	2.539	2.861	19
20	1.325	1.725	2.086	2.528	2.845	20
21	1.323	1.721	2.080	2.518	2.831	21
22	1.321	1.717	2.074	2.508	2.819	22
23	1.319	1.714	2.069	2.500	2.807	23
24	1.318	1.711	2.064	2.492	2.797	24
25	1.316	1.708	2.060	2.485	2.787	25
26	1.315	1.706	2.056	2.479	2.779	26
27	1.314	1.703	2.052	2.473	2.771	27
28	1.313	1.701	2.048	2.467	2.763	28
29	1.311	1.699	2.045	2.462	2.756	29
inf.	1.282	1.645	1.960	2.326	2.576	inf.

Table

C-3   The F Distribution (Values of $F_{.05}$)

Degrees of freedom for denominator	Degrees of freedom for numerator																		
	1	2	3	4	5	6	7	8	9	10	12	15	20	24	30	40	60	120	∞
1	161	200	216	225	230	234	237	239	241	242	244	246	248	249	250	251	252	253	254
2	18.5	19.0	19.2	19.2	19.3	19.3	19.4	19.4	19.4	19.4	19.4	19.4	19.4	19.5	19.5	19.5	19.5	19.5	19.5
3	10.1	9.55	9.28	9.12	9.01	8.94	8.89	8.85	8.81	8.79	8.74	8.70	8.66	8.64	8.62	8.59	8.57	8.55	8.53
4	7.71	6.94	6.59	6.39	6.26	6.16	6.09	6.04	6.00	5.96	5.91	5.86	5.80	5.77	5.75	5.72	5.69	5.66	5.63
5	6.61	5.79	5.41	5.19	5.05	4.95	4.88	4.82	4.77	4.74	4.68	4.62	4.56	4.53	4.50	4.46	4.43	4.40	4.37
6	5.99	5.14	4.76	4.53	4.39	4.28	4.21	4.15	4.10	4.06	4.00	3.94	3.87	3.84	3.81	3.77	3.74	3.70	3.67
7	5.59	4.74	4.35	4.12	3.97	3.87	3.79	3.73	3.68	3.64	3.57	3.51	3.44	3.41	3.38	3.34	3.30	3.27	3.23
8	5.32	4.46	4.07	3.84	3.69	3.58	3.50	3.44	3.39	3.35	3.28	3.22	3.15	3.12	3.08	3.04	3.01	2.97	2.93
9	5.12	4.26	3.86	3.63	3.48	3.37	3.29	3.23	3.18	3.14	3.07	3.01	2.94	2.90	2.86	2.83	2.79	2.75	2.71
10	4.96	4.10	3.71	3.48	3.33	3.22	3.14	3.07	3.02	2.98	2.91	2.85	2.77	2.74	2.70	2.66	2.62	2.58	2.54
11	4.84	3.98	3.59	3.36	3.20	3.09	3.01	2.95	2.90	2.85	2.79	2.72	2.65	2.61	2.57	2.53	2.49	2.45	2.40
12	4.75	3.89	3.49	3.26	3.11	3.00	2.91	2.85	2.80	2.75	2.69	2.62	2.54	2.51	2.47	2.43	2.38	2.34	2.30
13	4.67	3.81	3.41	3.18	3.03	2.92	2.83	2.77	2.71	2.67	2.60	2.53	2.46	2.42	2.38	2.34	2.30	2.25	2.21
14	4.60	3.74	3.34	3.11	2.96	2.85	2.76	2.70	2.65	2.60	2.53	2.46	2.39	2.35	2.31	2.27	2.22	2.18	2.13
15	4.54	3.68	3.29	3.06	2.90	2.79	2.71	2.64	2.59	2.54	2.48	2.40	2.33	2.29	2.25	2.20	2.16	2.11	2.07

(continued)

Degrees of freedom for numerator

Degrees of freedom for denominator	1	2	3	4	5	6	7	8	9	10	12	15	20	24	30	40	60	120	∞
16	4.49	3.63	3.24	3.01	2.85	2.74	2.66	2.59	2.54	2.49	2.42	2.35	2.28	2.24	2.19	2.15	2.11	2.06	2.01
17	4.45	3.59	3.20	2.96	2.81	2.70	2.61	2.55	2.49	2.45	2.38	2.31	2.23	2.19	2.15	2.10	2.06	2.01	1.96
18	4.41	3.55	3.16	2.93	2.77	2.66	2.58	2.51	2.46	2.41	2.34	2.27	2.19	2.15	2.11	2.06	2.02	1.97	1.92
19	4.38	3.52	3.13	2.90	2.74	2.63	2.54	2.48	2.42	2.38	2.31	2.23	2.16	2.11	2.07	2.03	1.98	1.93	1.88
20	4.35	3.49	3.10	2.87	2.71	2.60	2.51	2.45	2.39	2.35	2.28	2.20	2.12	2.08	2.04	1.99	1.95	1.90	1.84
21	4.32	3.47	3.07	2.84	2.68	2.57	2.49	2.42	2.37	2.32	2.25	2.18	2.10	2.05	2.01	1.96	1.92	1.87	1.81
22	4.30	3.44	3.05	2.82	2.66	2.55	2.46	2.40	2.34	2.30	2.23	2.15	2.07	2.03	1.98	1.94	1.89	1.84	1.78
23	4.28	3.42	3.03	2.80	2.64	2.53	2.44	2.37	2.32	2.27	2.20	2.13	2.05	2.01	1.96	1.91	1.86	1.81	1.76
24	4.26	3.40	3.01	2.78	2.62	2.51	2.42	2.36	2.30	2.25	2.18	2.11	2.03	1.98	1.94	1.89	1.84	1.79	1.73
25	4.24	3.39	2.99	2.76	2.60	2.49	2.40	2.34	2.28	2.24	2.16	2.09	2.01	1.96	1.92	1.87	1.82	1.77	1.71
30	4.17	3.32	2.92	2.69	2.53	2.42	2.33	2.27	2.21	2.16	2.09	2.01	1.93	1.89	1.84	1.79	1.74	1.68	1.62
40	4.08	3.23	2.84	2.61	2.45	2.34	2.25	2.18	2.12	2.08	2.00	1.92	1.84	1.79	1.74	1.69	1.64	1.58	1.51
60	4.00	3.15	2.76	2.53	2.37	2.25	2.17	2.10	2.04	1.99	1.92	1.84	1.75	1.70	1.65	1.59	1.53	1.47	1.39
120	3.92	3.07	2.68	2.45	2.29	2.18	2.09	2.02	1.96	1.91	1.83	1.75	1.66	1.61	1.55	1.50	1.43	1.35	1.25
∞	3.84	3.00	2.60	2.37	2.21	2.10	2.01	1.94	1.88	1.83	1.75	1.67	1.57	1.52	1.46	1.39	1.32	1.22	1.00

Table C-4

The F Distribution (Values of $F_{.01}$)

Degrees of freedom for denominator	Degrees of freedom for numerator																		
	1	2	3	4	5	6	7	8	9	10	12	15	20	24	30	40	60	120	∞
1	4,052	5,000	5,403	5,625	5,764	5,859	5,928	5,982	6,023	6,056	6,106	6,157	6,209	6,235	6,261	6,287	6,313	6,339	6,366
2	98.5	99.0	99.2	99.2	99.3	99.3	99.4	99.4	99.4	99.4	99.4	99.4	99.4	99.5	99.5	99.5	99.5	99.5	99.5
3	34.1	30.8	29.5	28.7	28.2	27.9	27.7	27.5	27.3	27.2	27.1	26.9	26.7	26.6	26.5	26.4	26.3	26.2	26.1
4	21.2	18.0	16.7	16.0	15.5	15.2	15.0	14.8	14.7	14.5	14.4	14.2	14.0	13.9	13.8	13.7	13.7	13.6	13.5
5	16.3	13.3	12.1	11.4	11.0	10.7	10.5	10.3	10.2	10.1	9.89	9.72	9.55	9.47	9.38	9.29	9.20	9.11	9.02
6	13.7	10.9	9.78	9.15	8.75	8.47	8.26	8.10	7.98	7.87	7.72	7.56	7.40	7.31	7.23	7.14	7.06	6.97	6.88
7	12.2	9.55	8.45	7.85	7.46	7.19	6.99	6.84	6.72	6.62	6.47	6.31	6.16	6.07	5.99	5.91	5.82	5.74	5.65
8	11.3	8.65	7.59	7.01	6.63	6.37	6.18	6.03	5.91	5.81	5.67	5.52	5.36	5.28	5.20	5.12	5.03	4.95	4.86
9	10.6	8.02	6.99	6.42	6.06	5.80	5.61	5.47	5.35	5.26	5.11	4.96	4.81	4.73	4.65	4.57	4.48	4.40	4.31
10	10.0	7.56	6.55	5.99	5.64	5.39	5.20	5.06	4.94	4.85	4.71	4.56	4.41	4.33	4.25	4.17	4.08	4.00	3.91
11	9.65	7.21	6.22	5.67	5.32	5.07	4.89	4.74	4.63	4.54	4.40	4.25	4.10	4.02	3.94	3.86	3.78	3.69	3.60
12	9.33	6.93	5.95	5.41	5.06	4.82	4.64	4.50	4.39	4.30	4.16	4.01	3.86	3.78	3.70	3.62	3.54	3.45	3.36
13	9.07	6.70	5.74	5.21	4.86	4.62	4.44	4.30	4.19	4.10	3.96	3.82	3.66	3.59	3.51	3.43	3.34	3.25	3.17
14	8.86	6.51	5.56	5.04	4.70	4.46	4.28	4.14	4.03	3.94	3.80	3.66	3.51	3.43	3.35	3.27	3.18	3.09	3.00
15	8.68	6.36	5.42	4.89	4.56	4.32	4.14	4.00	3.89	3.80	3.67	3.52	3.37	3.29	3.21	3.13	3.05	2.96	2.87

(continued)

Degrees of freedom for numerator

	1	2	3	4	5	6	7	8	9	10	12	15	20	24	30	40	60	120	∞
16	8.53	6.23	5.29	4.77	4.44	4.20	4.03	3.89	3.78	3.69	3.55	3.41	3.26	3.18	3.10	3.02	2.93	2.84	2.75
17	8.40	6.11	5.19	4.67	4.34	4.10	3.93	3.79	3.68	3.59	3.46	3.31	3.16	3.08	3.00	2.92	2.83	2.75	2.65
18	8.29	6.01	5.09	4.58	4.25	4.01	3.84	3.71	3.60	3.51	3.37	3.23	3.08	3.00	2.92	2.84	2.75	2.66	2.57
19	8.19	5.93	5.01	4.50	4.17	3.94	3.77	3.63	3.52	3.43	3.30	3.15	3.00	2.92	2.84	2.76	2.67	2.58	2.49
20	8.10	5.85	4.94	4.43	4.10	3.87	3.70	3.56	3.46	3.37	3.23	3.09	2.94	2.86	2.78	2.69	2.61	2.52	2.42
21	8.02	5.78	4.87	4.37	4.04	3.81	3.64	3.51	3.40	3.31	3.17	3.03	2.88	2.80	2.72	2.64	2.55	2.46	2.36
22	7.95	5.72	4.82	4.31	3.99	3.76	3.59	3.45	3.35	3.26	3.12	2.98	2.83	2.75	2.67	2.58	2.50	2.40	2.31
23	7.88	5.66	4.76	4.26	3.94	3.71	3.54	3.41	3.30	3.21	3.07	2.93	2.78	2.70	2.62	2.54	2.45	2.35	2.26
24	7.82	5.61	4.72	4.22	3.90	3.67	3.50	3.36	3.26	3.17	3.03	2.89	2.74	2.66	2.58	2.49	2.40	2.31	2.21
25	7.77	5.57	4.68	4.18	3.86	3.63	3.46	3.32	3.22	3.13	2.99	2.85	2.70	2.62	2.53	2.45	2.36	2.27	2.17
30	7.56	5.39	4.51	4.02	3.70	3.47	3.30	3.17	3.07	2.98	2.84	2.70	2.55	2.47	2.39	2.30	2.21	2.11	2.01
40	7.31	5.18	4.31	3.83	3.51	3.29	3.12	2.99	2.89	2.80	2.66	2.52	2.37	2.29	2.20	2.11	2.02	1.92	1.80
60	7.08	4.98	4.13	3.65	3.34	3.12	2.95	2.82	2.72	2.63	2.50	2.35	2.20	2.12	2.03	1.94	1.84	1.73	1.60
120	6.85	4.79	3.95	3.48	3.17	2.96	2.79	2.66	2.56	2.47	2.34	2.19	2.03	1.95	1.86	1.76	1.66	1.53	1.38
∞	6.63	4.61	3.78	3.32	3.02	2.80	2.64	2.51	2.41	2.32	2.18	2.04	1.88	1.79	1.70	1.59	1.47	1.32	1.00

Degrees of freedom for denominator

Table									
C-5	The Chi-Square Distribution (Values of χ_α^2)								

d.f.	$\chi^2_{.995}$	$\chi^2_{.99}$	$\chi^2_{.975}$	$\chi^2_{.95}$	$\chi^2_{.05}$	$\chi^2_{.025}$	$\chi^2_{.01}$	$\chi^2_{.005}$	d.f.
1	.0000393	.000157	.000982	.00393	3.841	5.024	6.635	7.879	1
2	.0100	.0201	.0506	.103	5.991	7.378	9.210	10.597	2
3	.0717	.115	.216	.352	7.815	9.348	11.345	12.838	3
4	.207	.297	.484	.711	9.488	11.143	13.277	14.860	4
5	.412	.554	.831	1.145	11.070	12.832	15.086	16.750	5
6	.676	.872	1.237	1.635	12.592	14.449	16.812	18.548	6
7	.989	1.239	1.690	2.167	14.067	16.013	18.475	20.278	7
8	1.344	1.646	2.180	2.733	15.507	17.535	20.090	21.955	8
9	1.735	2.088	2.700	3.325	16.919	19.023	21.666	23.589	9
10	2.156	2.558	3.247	3.940	18.307	20.483	23.209	25.188	10
11	2.603	3.053	3.816	4.575	19.675	21.920	24.725	26.757	11
12	3.074	3.571	4.404	5.226	21.026	23.337	26.217	28.300	12
13	3.565	4.107	5.009	5.892	22.362	24.736	27.688	29.819	13
14	4.075	4.660	5.629	6.571	23.685	26.119	29.141	31.319	14
15	4.601	5.229	6.262	7.261	24.996	27.488	30.578	32.801	15
16	5.142	5.812	6.908	7.962	26.296	28.845	32.000	34.267	16
17	5.697	6.408	7.564	8.672	27.587	30.191	33.409	35.718	17
18	6.265	7.015	8.231	9.390	28.869	31.526	34.805	37.156	18
19	6.844	7.633	8.907	10.117	30.144	32.852	36.191	38.582	19
20	7.434	8.260	9.591	10.851	31.410	34.170	37.566	39.997	20
21	8.034	8.897	10.283	11.591	32.671	35.479	38.932	41.401	21
22	8.643	9.542	10.982	12.338	33.924	36.781	40.289	42.796	22
23	9.260	10.196	11.689	13.091	35.172	38.076	41.638	44.181	23
24	9.886	10.856	12.401	13.848	36.415	39.364	42.980	45.558	24
25	10.520	11.524	13.120	14.611	37.652	40.646	44.314	46.928	25
26	11.160	12.198	13.844	15.379	38.885	41.923	45.642	48.290	26
27	11.808	12.879	14.573	16.151	40.113	43.194	46.963	49.645	27
28	12.461	13.565	15.308	16.928	41.337	44.461	48.278	50.993	28
29	13.121	14.256	16.047	17.708	42.557	45.722	49.588	52.336	29
30	13.787	14.953	16.791	18.493	43.773	46.979	50.892	53.672	30

Glossary

Alternate hypothesis: The hypothesis that suggests an effect on the variable(s) being studied; the hypothesis the researcher is interested in.

Analysis of covariance: Also known as ANCOVA; a combination of *analysis of variance (ANOVA)* and *regression analysis* that checks if the population means for a dependent variable are equal across an independent variable, while controlling for the presence of *covariates*.

Analysis of variance: Also known as ANOVA; a statistical test that checks if the means for several groups are equal. It is used as a way to avoid the increasing probability of a *type I error* that comes with running multiple *t-tests*.

Association: A relationship between the variables being studied; when a change in one variable is related to a change in another variable.

Assumption of sphericity: An assumption of repeated-measures ANOVA that the difference scores of paired levels of the repeated measures factor have equal variance.

Bar chart: A graphical representation of data, most useful for data at the nominal or ordinal level of measurement; the data categories are on the horizontal axis, while the frequencies of each category are on the vertical axis.

Bimodal distribution: A distribution in which there are two modes.

Bonferroni correction: A method used to correct for *Type I errors* that can arise from multiple comparisons.

Boxplot: A chart that represents the distribution of data values; it also illustrates the quartiles and any outliers.

Box's M test: A method used to test the homogeneity of covariance matrices.

Categorical data: Data made up of categorical variables, which are variables that can only have a limited number of values.

Causality: When a change in one variable is known to produce an effect or change in another variable.

Central tendency: The propensity for quantitative data to cluster around a certain point value; measures of typical or average values in a set of data points.

Chi-square statistic: A statistic used to determine whether or not the distributions of categorical data values differ from one another.

Codebook: The window in SPSS that allows you to define the characteristics of your variables prior to data entry.

Coefficient of determination: A measure of the amount of variability in one (dependent) variable that can be explained by a second (independent) variable.

Confidence interval: The range of values within which an estimated point would be expected to fall.

Confidence level: The level of assurance a researcher has that the data from a study/studies represent true values.

Confounding variable: Any uncontrolled variable that can have an effect on the outcome of a study.

Construct validity: Whether or not a measurement tool actually measures the specific idea of interest.

Construct: An idea or concept of interest.

Content validity: Whether or not a measurement tool captures the elements of the variable of interest.

Contingency tables: A table used to display the frequency distributions of variables, often used to study the relationship between two or more categorical variables.

Continuous variable: A variable that can be counted and has an infinite number of possible values (i.e., every value on a continuum); variables measured at the interval and ratio level.

Correlation: A standardized measure of the strength and direction of the relationship between two variables.

Covariance: A measure of how two variables are related to each other, ranging from negative infinity to positive infinity; a covariance of zero indicates that there is no relationship between the variables.

Covariate: A variable that affects the dependent variable, but is not the independent variable (not the variable of interest). Also known as a covariable.

Criterion-related validity: Whether or not the measurements from a tool or test are similar to the measurements from other, already validated tools.

Crosstab analysis: Using a contingency table to study the relationship(s) between variables and focus in on the most significant relationships.

Data: The values of variables.

Data analysis menus: In SPSS, the menus that allow you to create statistical outputs; the Analyze and Graph menus.

Data cleaning: Reviewing a data set to ensure that the data are complete and free of errors prior to analysis.

Data definition menus: In SPSS, the menus that allow you to add or change data; the Data and Transform menus.

Data file: In SPSS, the program files that contain the data values being studied (extension .sav).

Data set: A collection of data.

Degrees of freedom: A measurement of the opportunities for variability in a given statistical calculation.

Dependent group: A group where there can be multiple values from a single source.

Dependent variable: An outcome variable that is affected or influenced by the independent variable.

Descriptive statistics: Statistics that summarize the data gained from a sample or a population such as central tendency and variation.

Discrete variable: Also known as categorical variable; a variable that can be counted, but only has a finite number of countable categories; variables measured at the nominal and ordinal level of measurement.

Effect: When changes in the independent variable result in changes in the dependent variable.

Effect size: The measure of the magnitude of the relationship or difference between two variables.

Efficacy: The effectiveness of a given intervention.

Enter method: The default method in regression analysis, when all of the independent variables are fitted into the regression model at the same time.

Evidence-based practice: Utilizing data from reliable, scientific studies in combination with clinical judgment and patient preferences to determine the best course of action.

External validity: The validity of a study based on whether or not its results can be generalized from the sample to the target population.

F-statistic: A test used with normally distributed populations to determine if the means of said populations are equal.

Factorial analysis of variance: Data analysis that studies the effects of two or more factors on the dependent variable.

Fisher's exact test: A method used to test the relationship between categorical values in instances where the sample size is too small to use the *chi-square test*.

Frequency distribution: A method for presenting data that includes possible values for a given variable and the number of times each value is present.

Generalizability: The accuracy with which results from a sample can be extrapolated to encompass the population as a whole.

Goodness of fit: A measure of how well a model fits a set of observations.

Group comparisons: Comparing group values, as opposed to individual values.

Hierarchical method: A method in regression analysis that utilizes blocks of independent variables (chosen based on importance), added one at a time, to see if there is any change in the predictability.

Histogram: A visual method for presenting data that is similar to a bar chart, but instead groups data points into intervals, rather than individual categories; most useful for showing the distribution of continuous data.

Hypothesis testing: Examining data to determine whether there is sufficient evidence to accept (or reject) a research statement.

Independent group: A group where the values cannot overlap with the values of the comparison group.

Independent variable: In a research study, the variable that the researcher manipulates and that affects the other variable(s).

Inferential statistics: Statistics that allow a researcher to generalize about a population based on the results from the sample.

Instrument: See *Tool*.

Internal consistency: A measure of whether or not items in the same test, which purport to measure the same variable, are consistent.

Internal validity: The validity of a study based on the proper demonstration of a relationship between the variables being studied.

Interquartile range: A measure of variability; the difference between the values at the 75th percentile and the 25th percentile of a data set.

Interrater reliability: The ability of a test or scale to provide consistent values when used by different people.

Kruskal–Wallis test: A nonparametric method of analysis used to compare more than two independent samples and see if the samples come from the same distribution.

Kurtosis: A measure of the peakedness of a distribution.

Levels of evidence: A ranking system used to determine the quality and strength of results from differing types of research studies.

Levels of measurement: The four different scales of measurement, used to differentiate types of data (and the statistical procedures appropriate for the data). They are *nominal, ordinal, interval,* and *ratio*.

Line chart: A visual representation of data that is useful for following changes over time or for finding patterns in the data.

Linear: Generally referring to the relationship of one variable to another, which resembles a line.

Logistic regression: A type of regression analysis that predicts a group membership in a categorical dependent variable with independent variables, which are usually continuous but can be categorical as well; called *binary logistic regression* when the number of categories of the dependent variable is two.

Mann–Whitney test: A nonparametric method of analysis used to compare two independent groups to determine if the samples come from the same distribution.

Mean: A measure of central tendency; the arithmetic average of all values in a data set.

Median: A measure of central tendency; the exact middle value (when ordered consecutively) of a data set.

Methods of least squares: An approach used in regression analysis to find the line that best fits the data with the fewest residuals.

Mode: A measure of central tendency; the most frequently occurring number in a data set.

Multimodal distribution: A distribution in which there are three or more modes.

Multinomial logistic regression: A logistic regression with a dependent variable that has more than two categories.

Multivariate analysis of covariance: Also known as MANCOVA; an extension of analysis of covariance that is used in cases where there is one or more dependent variable and there is a covariate(s) that needs to be controlled.

Multivariate analysis of variance: Also known as MANOVA; an extension of analysis of variance that examines group differences on a combination of multiple dependent variables

Multivariate: When a design examines two or more continuous, dependent variables.

Nonparametric: Any tests or statistics that do not rely on an assumption of normal distribution.

Nonrandom missing data: When the data that are missing appear to follow a specific pattern.

Nonrandom sampling: The selection of members from a population based on something other than chance, often used to make a study more feasible or when the population of interest is difficult to access. Types include *convenience sampling, volunteer sampling, quota sampling,* and *snowball sampling.*

Normal distribution: A distribution of data in which the data values are equally distributed around the center data point.

Null hypothesis: The hypothesis that suggests there will be no statistically significant effect on the variable(s) being studied.

Odds ratio: A descriptive statistic used in categorical data analysis that measures effect size (the strength of the association between two binary data values).

Omega squared: The effect size for one-way ANOVA results.

One-tailed test: A test of significance that looks for an effect in a particular direction (positive or negative).

Orthogonal planned contrasts: Also known as a priori tests; comparisons that are planned before analysis of data has begun because certain results are expected. Orthogonal planned contrasts help reduce increasing type I error that comes from multiple comparisons.

Outlier: Any data value that is outside of the expected range of values.

Output file: In SPSS, the files that contain the results of the statistical analyses, along with any error or warning messages (extension .spv).

Parameter: A characteristic of a population.

Parametric: Any tests or statistics that assume a normal distribution in the data values.

Partial correlation coefficient: A measurement that allows us to look at the true relationship between two variables after controlling for an unwanted variable that may be affecting the relationship.

Percentile: Where a data point falls within the data set; specifically, how many data values fall above or below a specific point.

Phi and Cramer's V: Descriptive statistics that report the strength of an association between two categorical variables.

Pie chart: A circular chart in which the sections are proportionally representative of the frequencies of specific values of the given variable. It is most useful for the nominal and ordinal levels of measurement.

Point estimates: Single values computed from sample data.

Population: All the members of a group of interest.

Post hoc tests: Comparisons made to data after analysis to determine which means are contributing the greatest amount of variance;

Power analysis: A procedure used to calculate the minimum sample size required to be able to detect statistical significance based on effect size, or to calculate the level of power, given a sample size.

Predictor variable: Another name for the independent variable.

Qualitative variable: Variables whose data values are nonnumeric.

Quantitative variable: Variables whose data values are numeric.

R-square: A statistical measure of how well a regression line approximates real data points.

Random missing data: When the data that are missing do not appear to follow any sort of pattern.

Random sampling: The selection of members from a population based solely on chance; all members of the population have equal likelihood of being selected. Types include *simple random sampling, systematic random sampling, stratified random sampling,* and *cluster sampling.*

Range: A measure of variability; the difference between the largest and smallest values in a data set.

Regression model: The model created via regression analysis.

Relative risk: A descriptive statistic that measures the probability of an event occurring if exposed to a specific factor.

Reliability: The measure of whether or not a test is able to consistently measure a given variable.

Residual: The difference between the observed data and the data fitted to the regression model.

Sample: A subset of a population under investigation; the results from research on the sample are used to extrapolate to the population as a whole.

Sampling: The act of selecting a sample from a population.

Sampling distribution: The distribution of a given statistic as derived from all possible samples of a population.

Sampling error: The discrepancy between a statistic computed from a sample and the same statistic as computed from the entire population.

Scatterplot: A visual representation of the relationship between two continuous variables.

Simple effect analysis: Statistical analysis that examines the effect of one variable at every level of the other variable, to confirm if the effect is significant at each level.

Skewed: When the data's mean is pulled to one extreme or the other; an absence of normal distribution in a data set.

Skewness: A measure of how symmetrical a distribution is.

Sphericity-assumed statistics: Repeated measures design statistics provided if the *assumption of sphericity* is not violated.

Standard deviation: The average amount that data values will vary from the mean; the square root of the variance.

Standard normal distribution: A distribution in which the scales have been standardized to be able to compare different distributions; the mean is equal to 0 and the variance is equal to 1.

Statistical power: The probability of correctly rejecting the false null hypothesis.

Statistics: The characteristics of a sample.

Stem and leaf plot: A visualization of continuous data that shows both frequency distribution and information on individual data values.

Stepwise method: A method used in regression analysis where variables are added to the model based on predetermined statistical criteria. The three types of stepwise methods are *forward selection, backward selection,* and *stepwise selection.*

Syntax file: In SPSS, files that contain programmable commands used to generate analyses beyond those available in the interactive windows.

***t*-test:** A method for comparing two means from a populations.

Test–retest reliability: The measure of a test's ability to consistently provide the same measurements across time.

Tool: A device for measuring data.

Two-tailed test: A test of significance that looks for an effect without concern as to the direction (positive or negative) of the effect.

Type I error: When the null hypothesis is rejected by mistake; the probability of rejecting a true null hypothesis.

Type II error: When the null hypothesis is accepted by mistake; the probability of not rejecting a false null hypothesis.

Unimodal distribution: A distribution in which there is only one value designated the mode.

Univariate: When a design examines a single, continuous dependent variable.

Validity: The extent to which a test measures the variable it is designed to measure.

Variability: How much the values for a given variable are spread over a given range.

Variable: A trait or characteristic whose value is not fixed and can change (either from subject to subject, or within the same subject over time).

Variance: A measure of variability; the average difference between the data values and mean of a data set.

Wilcoxon rank-sum test: See *Mann–Whitney test.*

Wilcoxon signed-rank test: A nonparametric test used to compare paired data from the same population.

Windows and general purpose menus: In SPSS, the File, Edit, View, Utilities, and Help menus.

***z*-score/standardized score:** A measure of how far above (positive value) or below (negative value) a score falls, as compared to the mean.

Index